PANDEMICS

Essential Issues

PANDEMICS

BY MARY K. PRATT

Content Consultant
Alexandra Stewart
Department of Health Policy
George Washington University

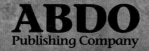

ABDO
Publishing Company

CREDITS

Published by ABDO Publishing Company, 8000 West 78th Street, Edina, Minnesota 55439. Copyright © 2011 by Abdo Consulting Group, Inc. International copyrights reserved in all countries. No part of this book may be reproduced in any form without written permission from the publisher. The Essential Library™ is a trademark and logo of ABDO Publishing Company.

Printed in the United States of America,
North Mankato, Minnesota
112010
012011

♻ THIS BOOK CONTAINS AT LEAST 10% RECYCLED MATERIALS.

Editor: Jill Sherman
Copy Editor: Paula Lewis
Interior Design and Production: Becky Daum
Cover Design: Marie Tupy

Library of Congress Cataloging-in-Publication Data
Pratt, Mary K.
  Pandemics / by Mary K. Pratt.
    p. cm. -- (Essential issues)
  Includes bibliographical references.
  ISBN 978-1-61714-776-0
  1. Epidemics--Juvenile literature. I. Title.
  RA653.5.P73 2011
  614.4--dc22

                          2010038064

TABLE OF CONTENTS

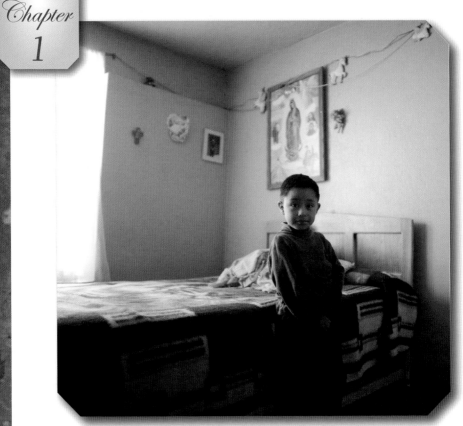

Four-year-old Edgar Hernandez was the first person known to have been infected with swine flu.

A New Threat

dgar Hernandez was an ordinary four-year-old boy until he became sick in spring 2009. In late March and early April, he experienced flulike symptoms, including a headache, fever, and trouble breathing. Edgar was given antibiotics and quickly recovered. For most children, that would have been the end of the story.

Edgar lived in the small town of La Gloria, Mexico, tucked into the rugged mountains of that country. A large number of residents in La Gloria became ill with flulike symptoms that spring. The Mexican government tested many of the sick residents and found that they had the regular, seasonal version of the influenza virus. But tests indicated that Edgar had something different. He had a new type of influenza. He became known as "patient zero"—the earliest individual known to have a particular disease.

This new strain, H1N1, was initially called the swine flu because it was first present in pigs. Then it spread to tens of thousands of people all around the world in a matter of months. In June 2009, the World Health Organization (WHO) announced there were nearly 30,000 confirmed cases in 74 countries. And

The World Health Organization

The World Health Organization (WHO) is part of the United Nations—an international organization of member countries founded in 1945. The WHO, formed in 1947, works to attain a high level of health for people in all parts of the world. It helps to fight diseases, especially infectious diseases, which can spread to other countries. The WHO often works with local health agencies that are dealing with an outbreak. They provide support to help treat patients and control the spread of disease. The WHO also monitors public health trends across the globe and promotes research for public health issues.

on June 11, 2009, Dr. Margaret Chan, the director-general of WHO, declared, "The world is now at the start of the 2009 influenza pandemic."[1]

PANIC AND BLAME

Even before WHO declared this new influenza virus a pandemic disease, fear set in among people around the world. Pandemic diseases are those that become widespread across a region or even the entire world. German Prime Minister Ulla Schmidt had expressed her concern in April when three cases of the H1N1 virus emerged in her country. "The development fills me with worry. None of us knows how far this will extend," she said.[2] That same month, the United States experienced its first H1N1-related death in Texas. Following news of the death, US President Barack Obama stated that schools might need to close as a precaution. He also announced that the federal government was preparing

WHO Declares a Pandemic

"No previous pandemic has been detected so early or watched so closely, in real-time, right at the very beginning. The world can now reap the benefits of investments, over the last five years, in pandemic preparedness.

"We have a head start. This places us in a strong position. But it also creates a demand for advice and reassurance in the midst of limited data and considerable scientific uncertainty."[3]

—WHO Announcement from Dr. Margaret Chan, June 11, 2009

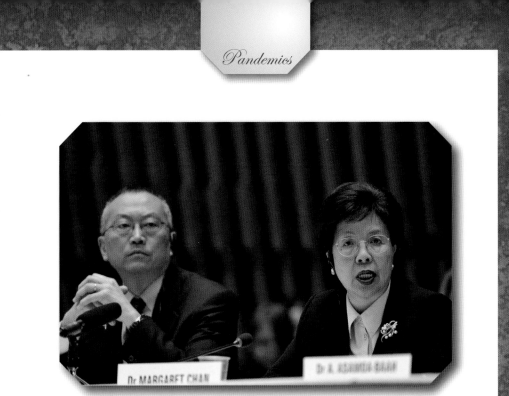

WHO officials announced new developments on the H1N1 influenza situation, at WHO headquarters in Geneva, Switzerland, in April 2009.

to deal with a possible epidemic, but there was "no cause for alarm."[4]

Mexico saw more disruptions. Schools and other public places were closed. Fearful residents wore surgical face masks to keep from catching or spreading germs. Some countries banned flights to and from Mexico. Meanwhile, the United States and other countries told their own citizens they should avoid traveling to Mexico.

Government officials around the world took steps to prevent the H1N1 virus from spreading. Angus

Nicoll, the influenza coordinator at the European Center for Disease Prevention and Control, stated,

> *The pattern at the moment is that of a mild disease, but one of the things that you've got to always remember with flu and particularly potentially pandemic viruses is that they have a nasty habit of changing and even becoming nastier over time. That's why in the EU, we're working so hard to make sure that the countries are prepared if this is going to get bad.*[5]

Some countries required airline authorities to report travelers who had flulike symptoms or scan international travelers for signs of influenza. Health officials said there was no evidence people got the virus by eating pork. Still, some countries banned imports of pork products from Mexico and US states that had reported H1N1 cases. The Egyptian government went even further and ordered as many as 400,000 pigs slaughtered in an attempt to stem the spread of the disease.

The panic harmed more than global trade and travel. It hurt people, too. In the United States, conservative talk-show hosts blamed Mexican immigrants living illegally in the United States for spreading the H1N1 virus and called for greater restrictions at the US–Mexican border.

US government officials, however, said that was not necessary. It would do little to stop the virus from spreading. However, such government reassurances did not stop the verbal assault on Mexican immigrants in the United States. "Illegal aliens are the carriers of the new strain of human-swine avian flu from Mexico. . . . If we lived in saner times, the borders would be closed immediately," radio show host Michael Savage said during his April 24 nationally syndicated show.[6] He also suggested that H1N1 could be a bioterrorist attack planned by radical Islamists.

The Poor Pig

A virus is a microscopic organism that needs another animal to survive and reproduce. Viruses often make their host animals sick, and sometimes viruses can be deadly. The viruses that cause influenza infect relatively few creatures. Pigs, some types of birds, and humans most often are susceptible to the influenza viruses. Influenza can easily mutate and move between these species. When a particular virus strain evolves from infecting animals to infecting humans, the name of that strain often reflects that migration. That was the case in 2009 as the pandemic influenza virus was initially called the "swine flu."

Like the virus itself, the name *swine flu* also underwent an evolution. It shed that moniker and was renamed in late April as the H1N1 virus. The US government led the efforts to change the name to the more clinical H1N1, which represents its genetic makeup. The change was made following concern from agriculture officials that the term *swine flu* was harming the pork industry. The H1N1 virus contains a mixture of genetic material from swine, bird, and human influenza strains.

A Year of Illness and Death

Because this virus struck young people disproportionately hard, many people became fearful for children. According to the US Centers for Disease Control and Prevention (CDC), half of the people who had confirmed cases of the H1N1 influenza during the first several months of the pandemic were 12 years old or younger. The CDC also reported that approximately 60 percent of known cases occurred in people between ages five and 24. Also, young people seemed to be developing the most serious cases of H1N1. According to the CDC, the median age of patients requiring hospitalization was 20. The median age of fatal H1N1 cases was 37.

Seasonal influenza is typically most dangerous to older individuals. Senior citizens make up 90 percent of the fatalities in any given year. By the end of 2009, scientists were still

Could H1N1 Come from a Single Farm?

Worldwide attention turned to the small Mexican town of La Gloria where the first known case of H1N1 developed. As H1N1 spread, the public was interested in tracking down exactly where the new disease developed. Some La Gloria residents and other advocates speculated that the new disease came from a nearby commercial pig farm, owned by the company Granjas Carroll de Mexico.

However, Mexican government officials said there was no evidence that the farm caused or contributed to the outbreak. The origins of H1N1 remain unknown.

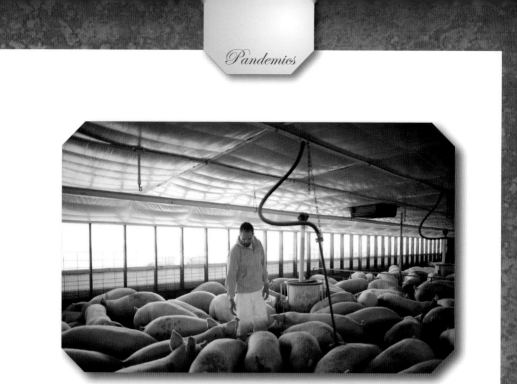

Some countries banned imports of Mexican pork after the swine-flu outbreak.

trying to determine why H1N1 hit young people with greater severity. Meanwhile, many people, regardless of age, found it difficult to obtain the recommended vaccine against the virus. Not enough vaccines were being produced to meet demand. The vaccine was intended to go to those who were most at risk first. But because of the pandemic, many people were fearful of contracting the disease.

By the end of the year, the WHO reported that more than 200 countries, territories, or communities had confirmed cases of the pandemic H1N1 virus.

The Global Influenza Surveillance Network

In 1952, the WHO organized the Global Influenza Surveillance Network (GISN) to monitor influenza viruses and alert global officials of pandemic potential. The GISN is made up of National Influenza Centers. These centers test samples taken from patients with influenza-like illnesses to determine whether an influenza strain made them sick. WHO Collaborating Centers analyze those samples. As of 2010, there were 134 centers in 104 countries.

Responding to Disease

Although modern medicine can successfully treat and prevent many diseases, infectious diseases have the potential to spread across the globe. As new diseases arise, medical professionals must be quick to develop vaccines and effective treatments. Governments must also act quickly to respond to a potential pandemic. They must encourage people to seek medical treatment, and in some cases, establish quarantines to prevent the spread of disease. With global travel, the modern world is susceptible to pandemic illnesses. Government agencies may choose to screen people arriving in their countries for illness. As germs continue to pose a threat to humans, modern medicine and social policy must be ready to fight back.

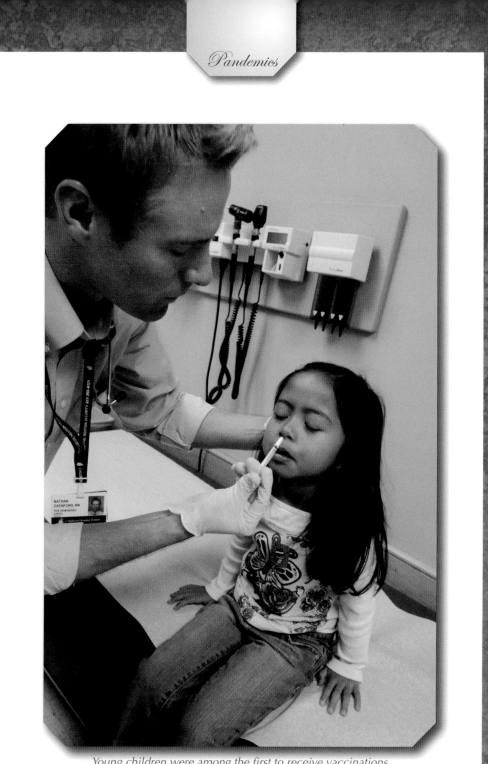

Young children were among the first to receive vaccinations for H1N1 influenza.

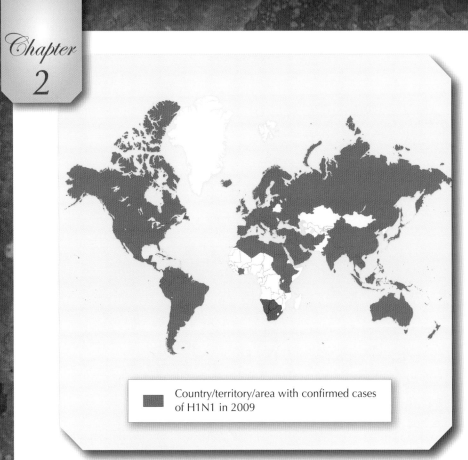

The H1N1 influenza became a global pandemic in 2009.

WHAT IS A PANDEMIC?

ven doctors, medical institutions, and government health agencies have no single, clear explanation of the word *pandemic*. "There is a lot of misinformation in the medical literature, and it is really quite hard to figure out what is and what is not a pandemic," said Dr. David M. Morens, an epidemiologist at the National Institute of Allergy and Infectious Diseases.[1]

In general, a pandemic is declared when many people in several different regions of the world have the same disease around the same time. A pandemic is a larger version of an epidemic, which happens when a communicable disease sickens many people around the same time in a small area. An epidemic that spreads around a large part of the world or sickens a high percentage of the population is a pandemic.

However, a disease does not have to be present in every country—or even most countries—to be considered a pandemic. The disease does not even have to be particularly deadly, either.

Controversy over Definition

It is important that the definition created by the WHO be accurate because it affects how governments, institutions, health officials, and the public react to an outbreak.

The WHO uses a six-point system, which was created in 2005, to alert governments around the world to the severity of a potential pandemic. The system describes how widespread an infectious disease has become. In Phase I, the disease being monitored occurs only in animals, and humans are not affected. As humans become infected and the disease becomes more widespread, it becomes a greater threat. By Phase 6, the disease has caused outbreaks in several countries and in multiple regions of the world. It has become a pandemic disease.

But some criticized WHO's definition of an influenza pandemic as too broad. According to Dr. Peter Gross, an infectious disease specialist at the Hackensack University Medical Center in New Jersey, under the WHO definition, some seasonal influenza viruses

Outbreak, Epidemic, or Pandemic?

Although the terms *outbreak, epidemic,* and *pandemic* are related, and some might think the words are interchangeable, each has a different definition.

An outbreak is when an endemic disease, a disease that is always present in an area or region, starts to infect a wider number of people in a particular region. It can often signal the start of an epidemic.

During an epidemic, a disease spreads quickly to a large number of people in a region or country, sickening them at the same time. A disease that is new to an area, or a new version of an existing disease, could cause an epidemic. A disease that is common in a region but strikes an unusually high number of people at a particular time might also cause an epidemic.

A pandemic is a version of an epidemic on a larger scale. An epidemic that spreads to multiple countries around a large part of the world at the same point in time is a pandemic.

could be incorrectly classified as pandemics. Seasonal influenza occurs every year. Although the strain changes each year, medical professionals are prepared for the disease, and vaccines are ready in advance to prevent infection.

Also, WHO's system does not take into account the potential mortality rate of the pandemic disease. Because the H1N1 virus was less deadly than other pandemic diseases, some governments believed WHO's system created unnecessary panic. Many people believed the H1N1 virus was incredibly dangerous. Some parents were afraid to send their children to school. Others were demanding that a vaccine be prepared immediately. Many governments believe that the severity of the illness should be considered, not just how widespread the infection is.

WHO Guidelines for Pandemics

In its Pandemic Influenza Preparedness and Response guidelines, the WHO outlines the phases of pandemic influenza. The guidelines outline six phases to a pandemic alert.

During Phases 1–3, an influenza virus is known to be circulating among animals, but there are few human infections. However, health officials must be watchful. Once human-to-human transmission has occurred, the virus has the potential to cause outbreaks. During Phase 4, human-to-human transmission of an influenza virus is common. The virus has caused sustained community outbreaks. By Phases 5 and 6, the virus has reached pandemic levels. Outbreaks have occurred in multiple countries in Phase 5 and multiple regions of the world in Phase 6.

Paul Zimmet spoke at the 2006 International Congress on Obesity in
Sydney, Australia.

REDEFINING PANDEMIC

As the H1N1 virus spread throughout 2009,
WHO officials found it necessary to revisit how they
defined an influenza pandemic. For many years,
the WHO defined an influenza pandemic simply as
causing "enormous numbers of deaths and illness."[2]
But according to its Web site at the end of 2009,

> *a pandemic is a worldwide epidemic of a disease. An
> influenza pandemic may occur when a new influenza
> virus appears against which the human population has
> no immunity. . . . Pandemics can be either mild or severe*

in the illness and death they cause, and the severity of a pandemic can change over the course of that pandemic.[3]

It is important for the WHO to have an accurate and effective definition of a pandemic. The WHO is considered an authority on global health issues. Its recommendations shape the response of local governments in fighting outbreaks of disease. Governments and health officials must react quickly if they are to control a potential threat to public health. They must research treatments, procure medicine, train medical personnel about the disease, and design systems for responding to local outbreaks. If the pandemic illness is potentially deadly, the response will need to be even more aggressive.

NONINFECTIOUS PANDEMICS

The influenza virus and other infectious diseases, such as smallpox,

The Pandemic Severity Index

In order to help communities prepare and respond to a pandemic, the US Department of Health and Human Services (HHS) announced a Pandemic Severity Index (PSI) in February 2007.

The PSI ranks pandemics from category 1 to category 5. Category 1 represents a moderate severity, while category 5 represents the most severe. The HHS said the severity of the pandemic would be determined by the percentage of infected people who die. Government and health officials could use the categories to help determine what actions a community needs to take in order to reduce the spread of the disease. Possible recommended actions range from asking sick people to stay home from school and work until they are no longer contagious to closing schools and canceling public gatherings.

After the Pandemic

At the height of a pandemic, when the rate of infection is highest, it is said to be at its peak. Once the number of infections begins to drop off, the disease enters a post-peak period. However, there is still a possibility for the levels to rise again, creating a new wave of infections. Eventually, the level of infection will drop off and return to the levels seen before the outbreak in most countries.

typhoid, and cholera, have been the cause of pandemics throughout history. But doctors, researchers, and scientists have also started to use the term *pandemic* to describe medical problems not caused by infectious diseases.

Calling obesity a pandemic is one of the most prevalent examples of this. More than 1 billion adults around the world are overweight, and 300 million adults are considered obese. At the 2006 International Congress on Obesity in Sydney, Australia, chairman Paul Zimmet declared, "This insidious, creeping pandemic of obesity is now engulfing the entire world. It's as big a threat as global warming and bird flu."[4]

Many of the most infectious and deadly diseases have been eradicated in parts of the world, including the United States. But now, noninfectious diseases such as obesity are the major killers of the era.

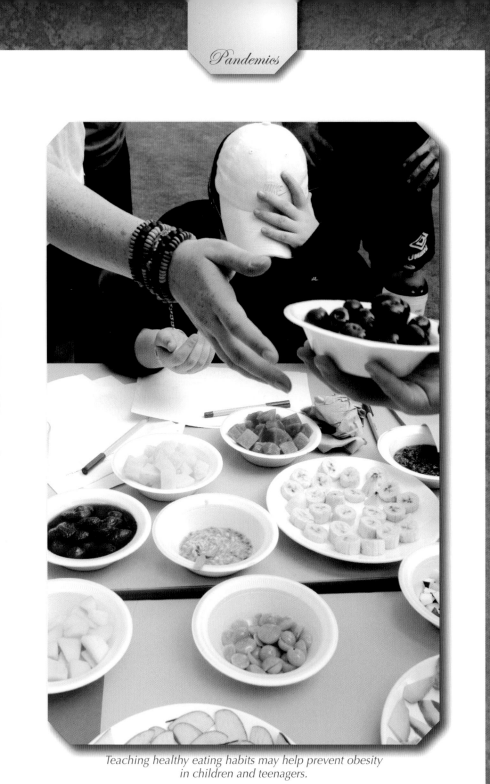

Teaching healthy eating habits may help prevent obesity in children and teenagers.

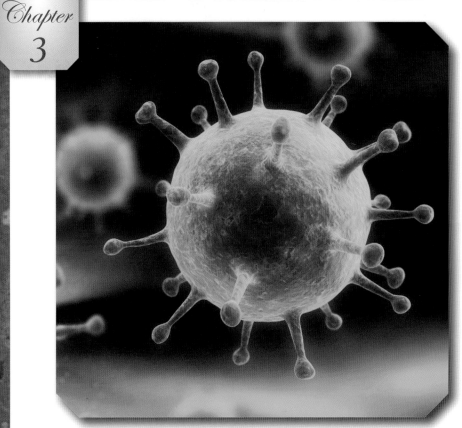

*Tiny microbes called viruses are responsible
for the spread of many diseases.*

WHAT CAUSES
A PANDEMIC?

The H1N1 pandemic started with a
microscopic organism called a virus.
One way to think of a virus is as a minuscule vessel
carrying genetic material. A virus cannot reproduce
on its own, so it must seek out a host. Once it

finds a host cell, the virus produces copies of itself. The host organism is now infected. Sometimes the host organism becomes sick as a result, and some viral infections can be deadly. The host organism can often spread the virus to others. Viruses may infect both plants and animals (including humans). Most viruses target specific species. The viruses that infect humans can cause a number of serious and deadly diseases, including AIDS, influenza, measles, polio, and smallpox.

Single-cell organisms called bacteria have also been responsible for a number of pandemics throughout history, including the bubonic plague, syphilis, and typhoid fever. Parasites, which are organisms that take their needed nutrition from their hosts, can also infect humans. Malaria, one of the most deadly pandemic diseases, is caused by a parasite. According to the WHO,

Early Treatments

Throughout much of history, doctors often knew less about treatments than they did about the diseases. As a result, the medical community turned to remedies that seem strange and, in some cases, dangerous today.

One remedy to ward off the bubonic plague, which devastated Europe during the fourteenth century, required sitting between two fires to purify the air. To treat syphilis, a sexually transmitted disease that reached pandemic proportions in Europe in the late fifteenth century, doctors used mercury, a dangerous toxin. During the 1918 influenza pandemic, some doctors suggested sticking a rag soaked in alcohol and chloroform into one's mouth or removing one's teeth and tonsils.

there were 247 million cases of malaria in 2008 and nearly 1 million deaths.

These disease-causing organisms can infect people in different ways. Many diseases are passed from person to person through the air. These germs are transferred when an infected person coughs or sneezes and someone else inhales the germs. Influenza, smallpox, and tuberculosis are transmitted this way. Some diseases are passed through more intimate contact, such as during sex, as is the case with HIV. Insects and animals can transfer disease to humans through bites. Bubonic plague, which caused millions of deaths in Europe during the fourteenth century for instance, was carried by fleas, which transmitted the disease to humans. The H5N1 strain of avian flu is passed from infected birds to humans. Most people contract the disease by

Quarantined at Ellis Island

Health officials have known for years that travelers often spread disease to new places. During the late 1800s and early 1900s, the US Public Health Service screened immigrants for disease before allowing them to enter the United States. Infectious disease was a serious problem, and the government did not want to risk an outbreak. Immigrants entering the United States passed through Ellis Island in New York where they underwent exams. If the doctors diagnosed a person with a communicable disease, the patient would be confined to the hospital for care and treatment. Often, this was the first time many immigrants had received such careful medical care. When they were cured of their illnesses, they were allowed to enter the United States.

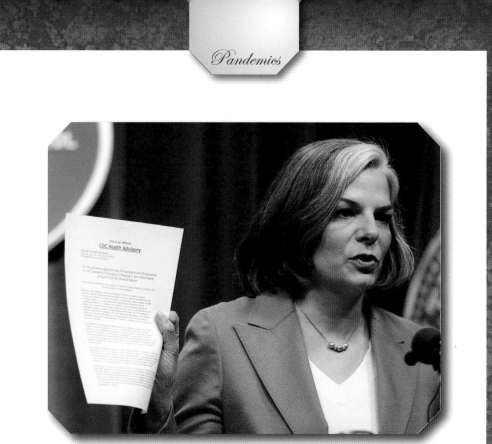

In 2006, CDC director Dr. Julie Gerberding warned the public of drug-resistant influenza.

handling infected poultry. This particularly deadly flu virus is rarely spread through human-to-human transmission.

EMERGING AND EVOLVING GERMS

The influenza virus does a very good job of spreading. It mutates easily and adopts genetic information from other viruses. Each year, the seasonal influenza virus is a slightly different strain, which is why researchers develop a new vaccine every year. This is also part of the reason the H1N1 strain became big news in 2009. It combined genetic material from swine, bird, and human influenza strains to create a new influenza virus. The influenza virus circulates in humans, but it is also present in pigs and birds. A strain that is present in animals does not always infect humans, but sometimes the virus will mutate and humans will become sick with a new strain of influenza.

When the H1N1 virus began infecting humans, no vaccine had been developed. Also, because it was new, most people did not have immunity against H1N1. The influenza virus is highly contagious. And because this new strain took medical professionals by surprise, they did not have an effective way to fight the disease. The conditions were right for an H1N1 pandemic.

The influenza virus is not the only disease that mutates. Other viruses change over time. Bacteria do as well,

Defining Diseases

• An infectious disease is caused by an external organism, such as a virus or bacterium that infects the body. It can be transmitted from one person to another.

• A noninfectious disease is not contagious and cannot be transmitted from person to person. Noninfectious diseases occur for a number of reasons, including genetic factors, environmental causes, and poor nutrition.

• Endemic diseases are continually present in a particular geographic area. Sub-Saharan Africa, for example, reports the most cases of malaria.

evolving for a number of reasons. For example, some bacteria have developed a resistance to the antibiotic medicines frequently used to kill them.

How Diseases Become Global

In part, modern lifestyles are to blame for creating conditions that are favorable for spreading germs around the globe. Travelers have always taken their diseases with them, infecting new populations. But today, travel is faster and easier than ever before. Because of increased international travel, diseases can spread from one region to another in a matter of hours or days. Many of the first cases of H1N1 diagnosed in the United States occurred in people who had recently traveled to Mexico, where the strain originated.

In addition, overcrowded cities contribute to the spread of disease. Cities ensure close contact between infected and uninfected individuals. People ride in crowded buses, wait in lines at restaurants and shops, and use public restrooms. All of these places have the potential to spread disease. That is why it is important to practice good hygiene and wash hands frequently, especially during flu season. This is also why people who are sick should stay home from school or work. They do not want to spread their illness to others.

Many of the conditions that have spread diseases and caused pandemics in the past are still at work today. Poverty continues to keep many people from getting medical care, which could contain an outbreak. Many times, sick individuals will not seek medical care because they cannot afford it. But if medical professionals do not know the population is becoming sick

International Traveler Triggers Fear

The potential health implications of global travel became clear in 2007 when an American man infected with multidrug-resistant tuberculosis flew from the United States to Europe and then to Canada. Multidrug-resistant tuberculosis is resistant to treatment by the two most powerful and commonly prescribed drugs to treat tuberculosis. It occurs when treatment of tuberculosis is interrupted and the levels of the drugs in the body are not enough to kill all of the tuberculosis bacteria.

Andrew Speaker and his wife flew to Europe on May 12, 2007. Speaker knew he was infected, and he had been warned against making the trip. Health officials in several countries tried and failed to prevent Speaker from traveling while infected. Speaker evaded authorities, and in order to return to the United States he traveled to the Czech Republic then flew to Montreal, Canada. He then traveled by car to the United States.

Public health officials feared that Speaker could expose dozens of people to multidrug-resistant tuberculosis, which could be fatal. Multidrug-resistant tuberculosis is just as contagious as regular tuberculosis, but it can be much more difficult and expensive to treat. Despite these concerns, Speaker traveled to multiple countries. His wife remained uninfected after the trip, and it is unknown whether Speaker infected others.

with an infectious disease, they may not learn of an outbreak until many people are already infected.

When people are vaccinated for diseases or treated for illnesses, there is also less of a chance for disease to spread. Doctors can advise those infected with a contagious disease on how to prevent spreading it to others. Depending on the severity of the disease, doctors may also advise individuals infected with serious illnesses to remain in hospital care. Medical professionals are also able to teach people about good hygiene and diets, which can keep them healthy. Many poor people are often unable to get adequate nutrition that could help them fight off an infection.

The lack of clean drinking water and sanitation services in many regions also contributes to the spread of disease. Such conditions are often exasperated by wars. For example, the African country Zimbabwe experienced a cholera outbreak in 2008 following the breakdown of its government. Cholera is an infectious disease that is transmitted through contaminated food and water. It causes diarrhea, vomiting, and dehydration, which can cause death in severe cases. The Zimbabwe outbreak occurred after interruptions to the

Travel Patterns and Disease

In the ongoing effort to understand how diseases are spread, researchers at Northeastern University in Boston, Massachusetts, used cell phone technology to track the locations of 100,000 people in Europe. The researchers found that the majority of people spent most of their time within the same ten-mile (16-km) radius. Approximately 2 to 3 percent of people traveled regularly over several hundred miles. The research, published in *Nature* journal in 2008, could be used to help prevent epidemics by better understanding human travel patterns.

country's water supply and sewage system. Overcrowding in cities also contributed to the severity of the outbreak. Zimbabwe saw nearly 100,000 cases of cholera and more than 4,000 resulting deaths in 2009.

Public health officials believe the world remains susceptible to pandemics—despite modern research and medicine. In 2010, the WHO warned that pandemic influenza may become a more common occurrence: "With the increase in global transport, as well as urbanization and overcrowded conditions in some areas, epidemics due to a new influenza virus are likely to take hold around the world, and become a pandemic faster than before."[1]

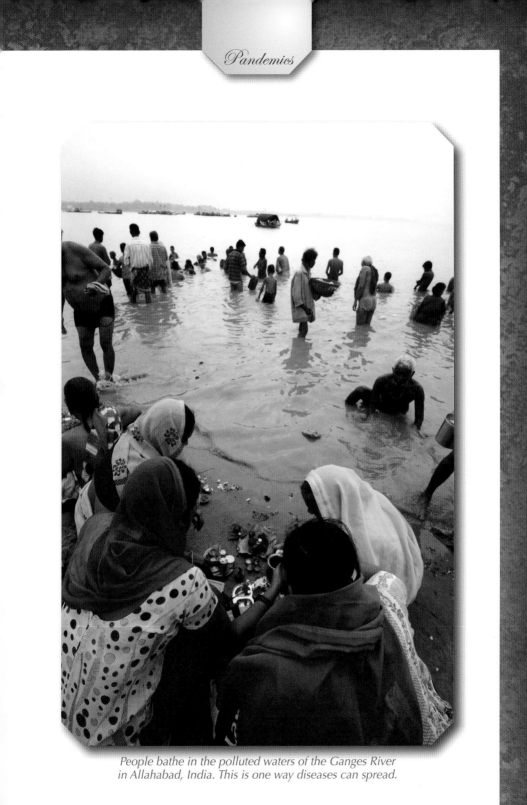

People bathe in the polluted waters of the Ganges River in Allahabad, India. This is one way diseases can spread.

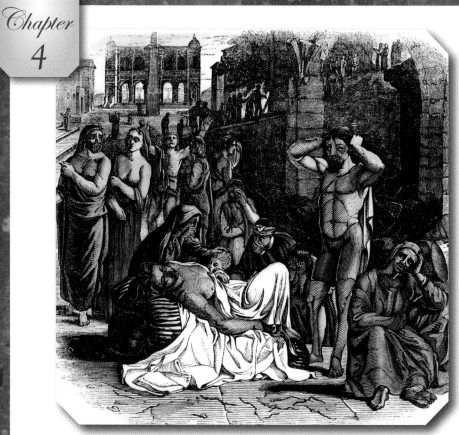

Plague victims are depicted in this woodcarving.

A History of Pandemics

he H1N1 flu pandemic of 2009 was just
one of many pandemics that have emerged
since the start of humankind. Some lethal germs
have existed for millennia. Others have mutated
into new strains able to survive modern medicine,

making them even more dangerous to humans. And sometimes, entirely new germs emerge, creating new diseases.

Early civilizations called widespread diseases "plagues" or "pestilences." Many people believed these events were punishments from deities. Others thought supernatural forces, such as demons or witches, had brought on the illnesses. But some ancient thinkers had more scientific beliefs. The Greek physician Hippocrates (circa 460 BCE–370 BCE) believed the environment caused illness. Modern researchers and scientists later identified tiny organisms called microbes as the cause.

Early societies understood the tremendous impact of pandemics. At times, ancient armies, including the mighty Roman army, were defeated not by opponents but by the diseases that spread rapidly among

Panic

Widespread disease incites fear and panic. Some Europeans blamed Jewish people for the bubonic plague pandemics of the fourteenth century, accusing them of poisoning wells and spreading the disease. Christians persecuted and tortured Jewish people during the hysteria that accompanied the plague. Christians in some parts of Europe similarly accused Jewish people for the syphilis pandemic that started in the late fifteenth century.

Others blamed the Catholic Church for the plague. They brought their loved ones to church and prayed for them, but they died anyway. Many monks and priests were becoming ill and dying as well. People began to think the plague had been brought to punish corrupt clergymen, and they blamed the church for bringing the plague to Europe.

the troops. Advancing armies were sometimes aided in their conquests by the diseases they carried unintentionally to their enemies. Some societies collapsed after too many of their citizens died.

BUBONIC PLAGUE

Bubonic plague was usually transmitted by fleas that fed on infected rats and then moved on to humans. The fleas transmitted the disease with their bite. Bubonic plague occurred repeatedly throughout history. Often unnamed by the civilizations of the time, it became known as the Black Death during the fourteenth-century pandemic. The disease likely earned this name because of the effect it had on the human body. Victims of bubonic plague developed large, swollen lymph nodes that were extremely painful. In severe cases, patients developed blood poisoning. This led to hemorrhages and gangrene in the skin and turned areas of the body black.

Typically, bubonic plague followed trade routes as the infected rats were often unknowingly brought along with traded goods. One of the first known occurrences of bubonic plague was the Plague of Justinian in the sixth century. Considered one of the

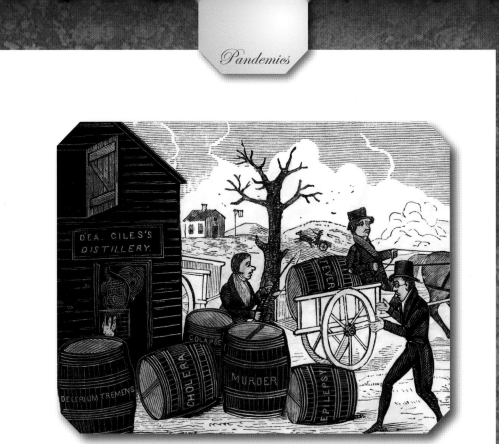

Europeans brought many troublesome diseases, including cholera, to the New World.

most devastating epidemics of all time, the plague cut the Mediterranean population in half over a period of approximately 60 years. It spread fear, death, and devastation through parts of the Middle East, North Africa, and Europe. By some estimates, it killed nearly half the people living in those regions.

After the Plague of Justinian, bubonic plague reached pandemic proportions again during the Black Death of the fourteenth century. Historians believe this devastating epidemic started in southern Russia. The disease spread from there, following trade routes to the Far East, the Middle East, and Europe. Historians estimate that one-quarter to one-third of the people living in Europe and the Middle East—or approximately 25 million people— died from the plague. The high death count led to widespread famine because there were not enough people left to raise food.

The Black Death changed society. With so many dead, local economies were devastated. Wages for skilled workers increased because there were fewer people who knew how to do the work. Some rural villages were completely wiped out by the plague. In response to widespread illness, public health became more important and many hospitals were established to treat the sick.

Eventually, the Black Death died out. But bubonic plague still exists. Many outbreaks of bubonic plague continued well into the 1800s, though without such devastating effects as the fourteenth century's Black Death. Today, bubonic plague occurs in all parts of the world with about 1,000 to 2,000 cases each year. Bubonic plague can be effectively treated with antibiotics, and all new cases are reported to local authorities so that preventative measures, such as rodent control, can be taken to stop the spread of the disease.

Syphilis

Syphilis is a sexually transmitted disease that became a pandemic in Europe in the late fifteenth century. This debilitating disease caused disfiguring skin lesions and led to infertility and insanity.

Some historians believe that sailors who traveled with Christopher Columbus became infected by native women in the New World and brought the disease back to Europe. Other historians believe syphilis could have been in Europe all along but that it had gone unnoticed until the pandemic. Pandemic syphilis quickly spread throughout Europe and into other parts of the world, including the Far East. Prostitutes, who serviced soldiers, often spread

Syphilis Had Many Names

During the pandemic that started in the late fifteenth century in Europe, syphilis was known by many names. It was called the great pox, distinguishing it from smallpox—another disease that killed many at that time.

Nationalistic leaders tried to place blame for the pandemic on other countries. They called it *morbus gallicus* (French disease) and *mala napoletana* (Neapolitan [Italian] disease). As the disease spread, it was known by similar names blaming German, Polish, and Spanish people as well. The Japanese called it the Chinese ulcer. The name syphilis finally emerged in Italy during the 1500s.

the disease. The soldiers then returned home and infected others.

This venereal disease swept through populations for hundreds of years. By the 1600s, syphilis was a major public health problem. It affected people from all social classes; there were cases among soldiers and prostitutes, nobility and royalty. The bacterium that causes syphilis was discovered in 1905, and an effective treatment was developed in 1909. But it was not until 1943 that penicillin was found to be a highly effective treatment for syphilis. Because of effective treatments for the disease and information on how to prevent sexually transmitted diseases, syphilis is much less common than it once was. However, the disease still occurs. In the United States, there are approximately 33,000 new cases of syphilis per year.

Cholera

Like many other diseases, cholera has struck often throughout history. Cholera is caused by the bacterium *Vibrio cholerae (V. comma)*. The acidity in stomach juices usually kills this bacterium. However, if someone ingests a large quantity of these bacteria, the bacteria may survive and enter the small intestine and multiply. The disease is further spread through water and food contaminated by cholera victims' feces.

Victims of cholera suffer from extreme cases of diarrhea, vomiting, and muscular cramps. They quickly become dehydrated and die. Death can occur in less than one day.

One outbreak, which began in India in 1826, lasted for 11 years. It spread through parts of the Middle East and Russia, eventually making its way to Western European countries, including England, France, and Austria. Immigrants traveling from Europe to North America brought the disease to Canada in 1832, and it soon reached the United States.

In 1863, another cholera pandemic spread out of India to the

Understanding and Defeating Cholera

Dr. John Snow, a surgeon, obstetrician, and anesthesiologist in England, is credited with first understanding how cholera spreads. In 1849, he published a paper suggesting that cholera was spread by contaminated water. Snow studied an area of London that was particularly hard hit by the cholera pandemic and determined sewage was seeping into a well that had been used by many of the victims. Public health officials were skeptical but agreed to remove the water pump's handle to make the water unavailable. No new cases emerged in the area.

Health officials in other countries were slow to understand such advances and usually resisted employing measures such as quarantines. They did not want to hurt businesses in the area by declaring quarantine.

East Indies and Asia. Muslim pilgrims from India carried the disease to the revered site of Mecca, located in modern-day western Saudi Arabia, and pilgrims in Mecca carried it back to their homes. Immigrants carried cholera to North America, infecting people not just in Canada and the United States, but also in the Caribbean and in South American nations as well.

As with other pandemics, the cholera pandemics of the nineteenth century brought not only suffering and death but panic and riots. Sometimes residents fled, leaving entire areas deserted as they tried to escape the disease. But these pandemics also gave rise to new understandings of the disease: what caused it and how it spread. This helped improve health and sanitation measures, which eradicated cholera from many parts of the world in the twentieth century.

Influenza

Influenza caused several pandemics during a 100-year stretch from the early 1900s to the early 2000s. The Spanish influenza of 1918 was one of the world's most devastating pandemics. The influenza killed more than 21 million people; some estimates are as high as 50 million deaths. Young, healthy adults were particularly vulnerable to the disease and suffered some of the greatest mortality rates of this pandemic. Just as past pandemics moved along trade routes, the 1918 influenza traveled along an expanded list of routes—railroad lines, shipping lanes, and military troop transports. Governments closed public places and canceled public events. In some cities and towns, there were not enough workers to handle even necessities, such as preparing the dead. Despite the deadliness of this pandemic, it was relatively short-lived, lasting only until the end of the year.

Two other significant influenza pandemics occurred later in the twentieth century. The 1957–1958 Asian influenza spread from China to more than one-third of the world's population. Just a decade later, another pandemic, the 1968–1969 Hong Kong influenza, emerged out of China and spread around the world.

SMALLPOX

Smallpox plagued human civilizations around the world for centuries. In the tenth century, Chinese doctors used a process called variolation to protect against smallpox. Variolation worked by infecting people with smallpox so they would develop a mild case of the disease. After they recovered, they were immune from developing the disease again. It was not until the late 1700s that British physician Edward Jenner developed a smallpox vaccine in Europe.

Still, even with these advances, the disease continued to infect millions of people even into the late twentieth century. In 1967, smallpox infected people in 43 countries around the world with an estimated 10 million to 15 million cases—including 2 million deaths annually. That year, the WHO set out on a campaign to eradicate smallpox. It dispatched medical teams whenever and wherever an outbreak occurred to vaccinate those in the area susceptible to smallpox until the disease disappeared. It took ten years, but the WHO achieved its goal. The last known naturally occurring case of smallpox occurred in Somalia in 1977.

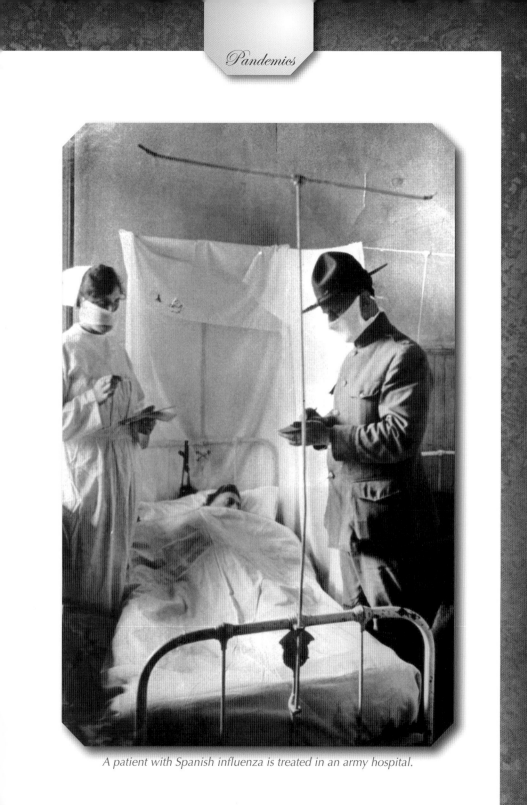

A patient with Spanish influenza is treated in an army hospital.

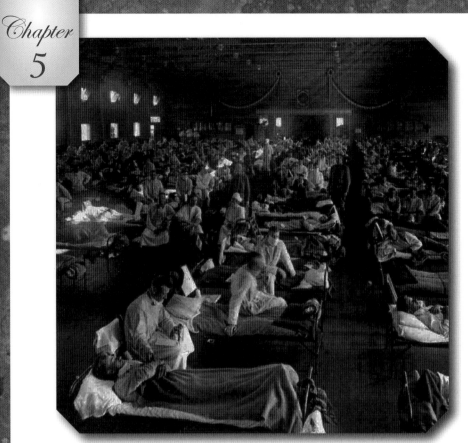

An emergency hospital near Fort Riley, Kansas, was filled with patients during the 1918 Spanish influenza pandemic.

Influenza Today

No country tracked the Spanish influenza of 1918. Some countries did not have a public health department that could monitor the disease. Those that did often did not require the influenza cases to be reported.

Civic leaders and public health officials, alarmed by reports of what was happening elsewhere, searched for ways to stop the disease from spreading. Some ordered schools, theaters, restaurants, and other public places closed. In some countries, people were required to wear face masks. But these measures did not stop the influenza virus from infecting millions of people worldwide.

By the start of the twentieth century, scientists understood that microscopic organisms caused disease and that some measures could successfully stop their spread. A major breakthrough occurred in the 1940s—the development of an influenza vaccine.

Still, the influenza virus continues to be of utmost concern to public health officials today. Seasonal influenza circles the globe annually and kills between 250,000 and 500,000 people. The virus is particularly difficult to fight, as it mutates every year, sometimes into a completely new strain to which humans have little or no immunity.

Spain and the Spanish Influenza

Despite its name, Spanish influenza does not appear to have started in Spain. However, Spain had the best records tracking the disease. The country had remained neutral during World War I and its health offices were better equipped to keep careful records of the outbreak.

ESTIMATED COSTS OF A PANDEMIC

Despite all the medical advances that occurred in the twentieth century, public health and influenza experts expected that future influenza pandemics were inevitable.

The threat of H1N1 has largely passed without major loss of life, but governments around the world still fear pandemic influenza because of the devastation it could bring. A pandemic could bring widespread worker absenteeism, lost economic productivity, and high medical costs.

Why Seasonal Flu Is Not a Pandemic

The seasonal flu, which is not considered a pandemic, kills 250,000 to 500,000 people worldwide every year. Yet the WHO declared a pandemic after 30,000 people worldwide died of the H1N1 virus. It raises the question: Why is the yearly seasonal influenza not considered an annual pandemic?

According to the US National Institutes of Health (NIH), seasonal influenza follows a predictable outbreak pattern. It occurs most often during the winter in moderate climates. In addition, many people have some immunity against each year's version from exposure to the previous year's influenza virus. Also, healthy adults are not usually at risk for serious complications. Instead, the very young, the very old, and individuals with health problems are most likely to face serious complications if they become sick.

Pandemic influenza is a rare occurrence. The NIH lists only three pandemic influenza outbreaks in the twentieth century. Also, the NIH considers influenza a pandemic when the population has no previous exposure to the virus strain and so has little or no immunity to it. Pandemic influenza also sickens healthy people at a greater rate and carries a greater risk for serious complications than seasonal influenza.

In 2008, the World Bank estimated, in a worst-case scenario, an influenza pandemic could kill 71 million people around the world and trigger a worldwide recession costing $3 trillion. Even a "moderate" pandemic would wreak havoc, according to the World Bank.

BEING PREPARED

A pandemic influenza virus today could spread more rapidly than in the past. More people are in contact with each other more frequently. Subway stations, airports, and athletic stadiums bring many people together in confined spaces. These places are good locations for diseases to spread. Also, more people travel globally and at greater speeds than at any other time in history.

Reaction to the H1N1 pandemic of 2009 showed how far the world had come in staving off a disaster. Governments around the world had public health departments that

Seasonal Flu Vaccine

The vaccine to prevent seasonal influenza can usually be prepared before an outbreak ever occurs. Because the influenza virus mutates very quickly, the vaccine from one year will not be effective the next year. Each year, different strains of influenza become more dominant and a new vaccine must be developed.

Health specialists meet annually to predict which strains are most likely to succeed and become the dominant form of seasonal flu. They are typically able to predict seasonal flu with great accuracy. This is important, because the decision about which strains of flu will be dominant must be made several months before the first outbreaks of seasonal flu in order to give vaccine manufacturers enough time to develop and produce the more than 100 million doses of vaccine needed each year.

were ready to implement their emergency plans to deal with the pandemic. They pushed for a speedy development of an H1N1 vaccine. They promoted practices that would slow the spread of the virus.

Avian Flu

In the 1990s, public health workers around the world were watching a particularly deadly form of the influenza virus: the H5N1 avian flu. The strain emerged in Asia in 1997. By the end of 2009, the WHO reported 467 cases worldwide. Although the number of cases seems minuscule, the mortality rate was staggeringly high. Out of those 467 cases, 282 died, for a mortality rate of 60 percent. The strain appeared to be passed from birds to humans who had close contact with infected fowl. Public health officials feared that a mutation could make human-to-human contact possible. If this had happened, a deadly influenza virus could have spread rapidly around the world.

US President Barack Obama, along with others, promoted the idea of frequent hand washing and staying home when ill as smart strategies for fighting the pandemic. Although there were an estimated 47 million cases of H1N1 in the United States by the end of 2009, only a fraction of those cases—about 10,000—resulted in death.

Still, the response to the pandemic was not fast enough for some people. Though researchers went to work on a vaccine shortly after the H1N1 outbreak, it still took them months to find a safe and effective vaccine. And even after the vaccine was discovered, it still needed to be produced on a large scale and distributed to populations all over the world.

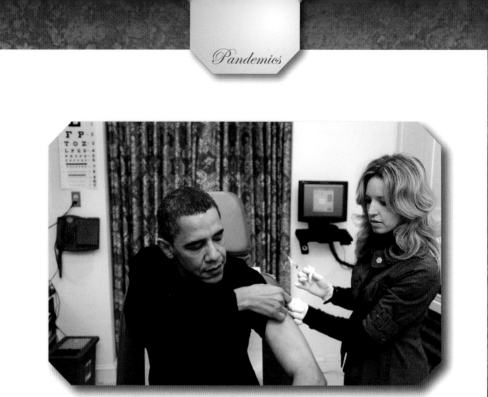

A White House nurse administered the H1N1 vaccine to US President Barack Obama.

By October 2009, the vaccine was being distributed to medical facilities for administration. But in many cases, not enough vaccine had been sent to meet the demand. Many people were turned away without getting vaccinated. The US government had predicted that 160 million doses would be ready by late October. However, because the vaccine required a longer than normal gestation period, only 30 million doses had been prepared. Priority for the vaccines went to those most at risk. Health professionals, individuals with compromised immune systems, and pregnant women were among the first to be vaccinated.

After the initial few weeks of vaccine distribution, more people were allowed to receive the vaccine. However, despite the initial outcry for more vaccine, by early 2010 the US government had a surplus of unused vaccine. Meanwhile, poor countries in Central Asia, Northern Africa, and Eastern Europe were being hit hardest by the H1N1 outbreak and were without adequate vaccine supply.

Public health agencies around the world continue to track potential and real pandemic viruses. Also, the WHO continually monitors the influenza virus through its network of National Influenza Centers around the world. Vaccines, along with antiviral agents and antibiotics, are widely available. However, they could become in short supply, along with other medical resources, during a severe pandemic.

Will County residents waited for the H1N1 vaccine at a high school in Plainfield, Illinois, in October 2009.

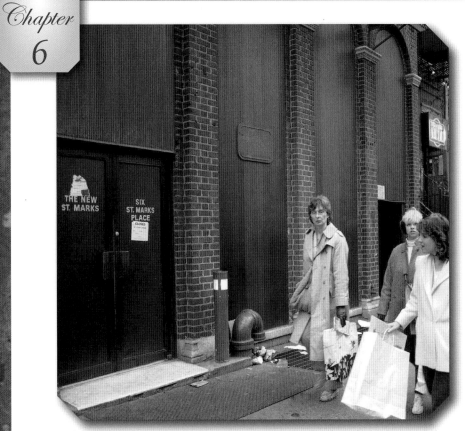

In 1986, St. Mark's Baths in New York, along with other places frequented by gay men, was closed in an attempt to prevent the spread of AIDS.

HIV/AIDS

The first signs of the Acquired Immune Deficiency Syndrome, or AIDS, pandemic appeared in the summer of 1981. In June, the CDC published a brief clinical report that showed five young men in the Los Angeles area had a rare form of pneumonia called Pneumocystis carinii pneumonia (PCP). The CDC also noted that all five men were homosexual. Two months later, the CDC reported that since 1980, more than 100 homosexual men had been diagnosed with either PCP or a rare cancer called Kaposi's sarcoma (KS). In some cases, men had been diagnosed with both diseases. The CDC investigated these unusual cases, trying to determine the cause. Meanwhile, the number of cases grew exponentially.

The patients were infected with a new disease called AIDS. The cause of death in the early cases was KS or PCP, but early AIDS patients were diagnosed with a number of serious infections, including lymphomas and cancers. In late 1982, researchers were able to identify those at greatest risk for getting the disease: homosexual or bisexual men, intravenous drug users,

Homosexuals, AIDS, and the Public

HIV, the virus that causes AIDS, primarily infected homosexual men in the United States in the early years of the disease. Because of that, the sexual practices in the gay community became a topic of public health interest. Gay men also became the center of a political and societal debate.

Some advocates pushed to close gay bars and restaurants frequented by gay men. Others argued that such moves were a violation of civil rights. Some also blamed the homosexual community for AIDS and called the disease God's punishment against gays.

hemophiliacs, and Haitians. But some patients
did not fit into any of these four groups. Patients
suffered from severe pain, and the cost to treat each
patient was approximately $64,000; the hospital
bills from the first 300 cases totaled $18 million.

Doctors, epidemiologists, infectious-disease
specialists, and public health officials tried to
explain how AIDS was transmitted. But they could
not account for how all the victims developed the
symptoms. Also in late 1982, more than two dozen
infants and children were infected. Researchers also
reported numerous cases in major cities, including
Miami, New York City, and San Francisco as well as
cities outside the United States.

By the end of 1982, the CDC determined that
AIDS could be transmitted from one person to
another through blood. Researchers also rightly
suspected that it was passed during sexual contact.

Scientists also theorized how AIDS developed.
Many believed that it originated in Central Africa.
AIDS resembled a disease present in chimpanzees
there. If a similar disease existed in primates, it
could have been transferred to humans.

As the awareness of the existence of AIDS grew,
so did the public's fear and misunderstanding of

this incurable and fatal disease. People wondered whether it could be spread through casual encounters—holding or shaking hands with someone who was infected, for example, or through insect bites. Doctors, nurses, and other health-care workers feared they could get AIDS when working with patients or through an accidental prick of a needle used on an AIDS patient.

PREVENT, TREAT, AND CURE

Fear of AIDS transmission gave rise to new

Fear Overrules Empathy

When AIDS first emerged, many people were fearful that they could become infected with the disease. AIDS was often poorly understood by the public. People's fear often manifested as prejudice. Patients were ostracized for being sick. Children were also sometimes the targets of that fear during the early years of the AIDS pandemic.

This issue came to the forefront in the United States when Ryan White, an Indiana teenager who had contracted AIDS through a blood transfusion, was barred from attending school in 1985. He and his mother, Jeanne White, fought the decision and got a court order forcing Western Middle School in Kokomo, Indiana, to admit him.

White's case was not unique. Parents of children with AIDS in other towns and cities had similar problems. School officials and parents were fearful that other children would contract the disease through casual contact.

But Ryan and his mother fought back with education. They told their story to the national media, and they provided information about HIV and AIDS. Ryan White died in April 1990. He had become well known for his activism. In August of that same year, Congress enacted the Ryan White Comprehensive AIDS Resources Emergency (CARE) Act to improve the quality and availability of care for low-income, uninsured, and underinsured HIV patients.

practices. Health-care workers and emergency responders started wearing protective gloves to prevent the spread of AIDS. The process of collecting blood used for transfusions changed as well. Donated blood needed to be screened for AIDS to prevent accidental transmission to patients. Public health campaigns promoted the message of "safe sex," that is, using condoms to decrease the risk of transmitting AIDS.

As AIDS spread worldwide, the need for prevention practices became more important. But these practices were not always quickly adopted. Some people questioned the science behind this new epidemic. Others were unwilling to bring about new practices for social, political, and financial reasons. AIDS also sparked renewed debate about public health policies. Some advocated for measures such as reporting infected individuals to public health officials. Others promoted measures such as providing free, clean needles to illegal drug users.

As these protective measures developed, researchers continued to learn more about the disease and the virus that causes it. In 1983, American and French researchers working independently identified the virus that causes

AIDS. It became known as human immunodeficiency virus, or HIV. The discovery of HIV opened up new possibilities for prevention and treatment.

HIV infects white blood cells, which play a role in the immune system. The virus tells the infected cells to produce more HIV, spreading the disease. Eventually, the white blood cells will die. Although people may be infected with HIV, they may never develop AIDS. Patients with HIV develop AIDS when their white blood cell counts drop to 200 cells per microliter of blood. With treatment, they may later be able to increase their white blood cell counts above that mark. However, people who are diagnosed with AIDS are considered to have AIDS even if their white blood cell counts increase.

What Is a Retrovirus?

HIV is a retrovirus. A retrovirus is a type of virus that stores its genetic information as RNA. RNA carries the information stored in DNA. Most other viruses, along with most other living organisms, store their genetic information in DNA. A retrovirus uses RNA to insert a copy of its DNA into a healthy cell. When the host cell replicates itself, it also replicates the virus's DNA. This is how retroviruses spread in the body.

A New Preparedness

When the AIDS pandemic began in the early 1980s, people with the disease usually died from

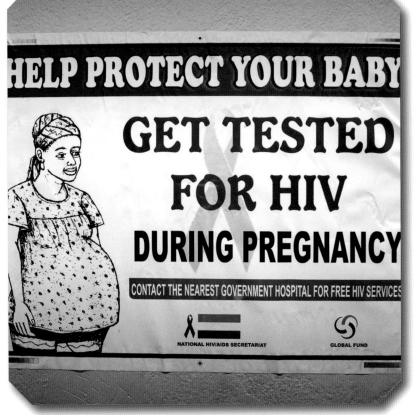

*Health education and safe sex methods are promoted
to inform the public about AIDS.*

it. The AIDS virus weakens the immune system,
the body's defense system against infection and
disease. This makes patients infected with AIDS
more susceptible to other diseases. AIDS patients
usually develop other diseases including pneumonia,

infections of the esophagus, Kaposi's sarcoma, and tuberculosis. People with AIDS may contract several of these diseases. Typically, people with AIDS will die not from the AIDS virus itself but from complications due to the many other diseases they become infected with because of AIDS.

During the 1980s, treatments for people with AIDS typically addressed these other illnesses, which doctors were more familiar with. However, there were no specific treatments to slow the progression of AIDS. Researchers quickly began working on a treatment for AIDS. During the three decades following the emergence of AIDS, researchers developed antiretroviral drugs and other treatments that greatly improved the quality of life and chances of survival for those diagnosed with HIV. But these drugs carried a hefty price: $10,000 to $12,000 a year in the United States.

Both a cure and a vaccine still remain elusive. Scientists continue to develop more effective drugs that are better tolerated by patients. Public health officials continue to educate society on the importance of safe sex and other preventative measures.

Hope for a Vaccine

The WHO estimates that nearly 35 million people worldwide had HIV in 2008. In addition, an estimated 2.7 million new cases of HIV were diagnosed that year. Approximately 2 million people around the world died that year due to AIDS. Sub-Saharan Africa experienced the highest number of cases—22.4 million. South and Southeast Asia had the second-highest number with 3.8 million cases.

AIDS is especially devastating in many parts of Africa. More than 30 percent of adults in sub-Saharan Africa are infected with AIDS, and life expectancy there is only 47 years old. Many children have parents with AIDS. As children attempt to care for their sick parents, their education often suffers. Because many adults are dying young from AIDS, their children become orphans, some of

Discounting Drugs to Developing Countries

In the early twenty-first century, drug companies came under pressure to provide lifesaving drugs for HIV and AIDS patients in African and Caribbean countries at steeply discounted prices. Developing countries, particularly those in Africa, were among the hardest hit by the AIDS pandemic. But they were the least able to afford the costly drugs, which can significantly extend and improve the quality of an HIV/AIDS patient's life. Drug companies from Europe, the United States, and other countries agreed to cut prices. But the cost of drugs in developing countries remains an important issue in international circles.

whom are infected with AIDS themselves. In South Africa, an estimated 70,000 babies are born with HIV every year.

One of the reasons HIV/AIDS is so prevalent in these regions is because of poor health care and lack of information about preventing sexually transmitted diseases. Safe sex practices, the use of condoms in particular, can do a great deal to prevent the spread of HIV. However, condom distribution is often insufficient to effectively combat the problem, with approximately four to ten condoms being distributed per male per year.

People in regions devastated by AIDS are least likely to be able to afford the high cost of the drugs for AIDS treatment. The drugs are also difficult to obtain, and in some countries, such as South Africa, government leaders have told people the drugs are ineffective. Therefore, the large majority of people with HIV/AIDS in Africa go without treatment. AIDS has a financial toll on society in Africa and Asia as well. Mortality among adults means fewer workers, fewer farmers, and fewer parents to help raise children.

An effective vaccine against HIV would go a long way in preventing the spread of AIDS. Medical

The Pandemic and Its Orphans

The WHO estimated that in 2007 approximately 15 million children lost one or both parents to AIDS, including nearly 12 million children in sub-Saharan Africa. The number of orphans in Africa was expected to grow to 18 million by 2010. International agencies try to help care for these children, but many still end up fending for themselves. Some become forced laborers, and others are abused. Orphans sometimes live in the wild or with a grandparent who does not have enough money to care for them. Some children are lucky enough to find help in orphanages or with agencies that find them new homes.

researchers continue to investigate the problem with little success. In 2009, Thai scientists announced some promising results for a trial of their HIV vaccine. However, even if this vaccine proves to be viable, it will still take years before it is ready for distribution.

"AIDS continues to be a major global health priority," the WHO stated in its 2009 AIDS epidemic update. "AIDS-related illnesses remain one of the leading causes of death globally and are projected to continue as a significant global cause of premature mortality in the coming decades."[1]

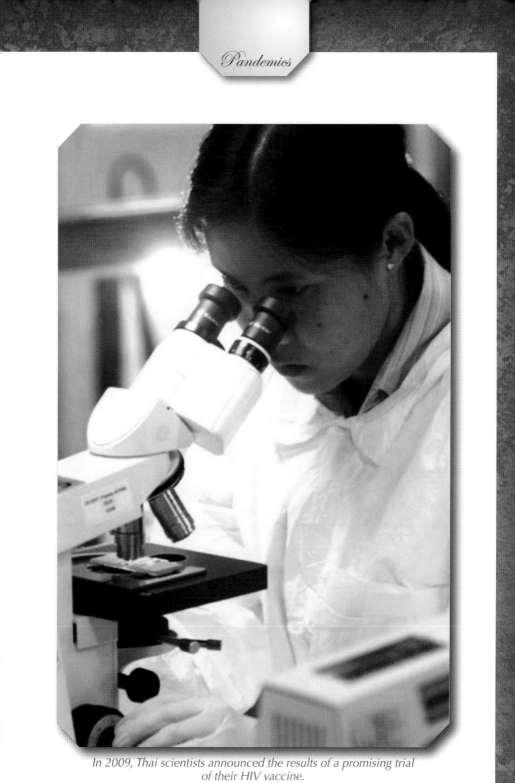

In 2009, Thai scientists announced the results of a promising trial
of their HIV vaccine.

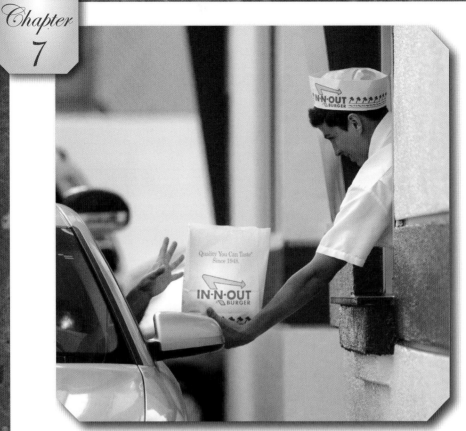

High-fat diets and sedentary lifestyles are largely to blame for the increase in obesity rates.

THE RISE OF THE OBESITY PANDEMIC

*D*uring the latter part of the twentieth century, researchers saw that obesity was affecting people around the world in greater numbers than ever before. Its rapid increase and its geographic reach were significant.

The WHO identified a primary cause: "increased consumption of more energy-dense, nutrient-poor foods with high levels of sugar and saturated fats, combined with reduced physical activity."[1] In North America, the United Kingdom, Eastern Europe, the Middle East, the Pacific Islands, Australasia, and China, obesity rates have more than tripled since 1980. And obesity rates are increasing markedly in developing nations as well. According to the WHO, there were more than 1 billion overweight adults by 2010 and at least 300 million of them were obese.

But like other pandemics, this one did not strike with equal force everywhere. WHO statistics show that obesity levels ranged from less than 5 percent in China, Japan, and some African countries to more than 75 percent in urban areas of Samoa in the South Pacific.

Obesity is not an infectious disease. It is not contagious in the way that many other pandemic diseases, such as influenza, are. Rather,

Defining Obesity

The body mass index, or BMI, measures an individual's body fat based on height and weight. It has become a common way to assess obesity. BMI is only a quick way to see if a person may be overweight, however. Because it does not take a person's muscle mass into account, muscular individuals may be inaccurately categorized as obese using BMI. A more extensive test to calculate a person's percentage of body fat gives a more accurate measurement.

"overweight and obesity result from an energy imbalance."[2] In simple terms, the body takes in more calories than it burns through physical activity.

However, many factors can influence an individual's propensity to gain weight beyond how much he or she eats and exercises. An individual's genes help determine the likelihood of that person gaining excess weight. Genes also determine how fast the body burns energy. But the rapid increase in obesity cases stemmed primarily from societal developments that occurred in the twentieth century. More people began to switch to diets that had more fats and sugars. Poor people tended to eat less nutritiously because access to high-calorie, low-nutrition foods became increasingly affordable. People also moved away from jobs that required physical labor. People's lives became more sedentary at work and home. More people owned cars, which further cut down on physical activity.

"Change starts with the individual choices we as Americans make each day for ourselves and those around us. Balancing good nutrition and physical activity while managing daily stressors is always a challenge, but one that can be achieved. Finding time to shop for and prepare healthy meals after work and between family activities requires planning. . . . Eating excess calories contributes to obesity, but so does watching too much television and sitting for hours in front of a computer."[3]

—US Surgeon General Regina Benjamin, MD, PhD

But as global obesity has increased, researchers have started to examine other factors. For example, evolutionary factors may play a role in increased obesity. Bacteria living in the human digestive system encourage the body to store energy as fat and keep it on. This was useful in previous eras when food was not plentiful, but it could be harmful today when food is always available.

OBESITY'S IMPACT

Obesity has a tremendous impact on an individual's health and well-being. An obese individual has a 50 to 100 percent increased risk of premature death compared to someone who is not overweight. An estimated 300,000 deaths each year are attributable to obesity. Obese individuals face other health problems as well. They have an increased risk of coronary heart disease, type 2 diabetes, certain cancers, and a host of other diseases and disorders.

Associated Diseases

Obesity puts individuals at higher risk for a host of other diseases—some of which are life threatening. Those diseases include:
- Type 2 diabetes
- Heart disease
- Stroke
- Hypertension (high blood pressure)
- Gallbladder disease
- Osteoarthritis (degeneration of joint cartilage and bone)
- Sleep apnea (temporary stop in breathing during sleep)
- Asthma
- Cancer
- High blood cholesterol
- Psychological disorders, such as depression

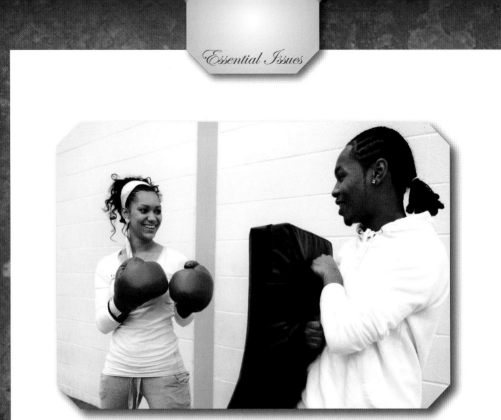

Healthy lifestyles that include exercise can help teens maintain a healthy weight.

Society also pays a price for this pandemic. Consider, for example, how much obesity impacts the US health-care system. According to the US Surgeon General's office, the total cost of obesity in 2000 was estimated at $117 billion. Those costs include doctor visits, medical tests, and prescription drugs. They also include the "value of wages lost by people unable to work because of illness or disability, as well as the value of future earnings lost by premature death."[4] Americans spend billions of dollars every year on weight-loss programs, ranging from self-help groups and books to diets and surgery.

The Fight against Fat

As the problem of obesity became pandemic, doctors, scientists, and public health workers started to devise new ways to fight this disease. In addition to advising overweight individuals to eat less and exercise more, they promoted changes aimed at slimming down society. They pushed for better nutrition labels on foods and more funding for research. They advocated for communities to create more recreational opportunities for their residents. And they lobbied for more nutrition and physical education for children and adults.

Efforts to combat obesity were global. In 2004, the WHO issued its Global Strategy on Diet, Physical Activity, and Health. The WHO seeks to address the obesity pandemic through increasing awareness about the role of diet and exercise in a healthy lifestyle and in reducing obesity. The WHO also plans to promote scientific research into the obesity problem to better understand how to deal with the issue.

The WHO also advocated for public policies that would allow people access to nutritional foods and opportunities for physical activity. WHO representatives asked for more programs and trained staff, who could provide obese people with support and advice to help them lose weight and prevent weight gain.

Childhood Obesity

Of even greater concern for many health professionals is the rise in childhood obesity. Childhood obesity is particularly problematic because obese children tend to stay obese as they grow. They are more likely to develop weight-related health issues such as diabetes, high cholesterol, and high blood pressure at younger ages. Childhood obesity is also linked to low self-esteem and depression.

Overweight and obese children are more likely than normal weight children to become overweight or obese adults. This means obese children are likely to have serious health problems throughout their entire lives.

In 2008, the CDC reported that in the United States approximately 18 percent of children ages 6 to 18 were obese. This was a sharp increase from 5 percent in 1980. But childhood obesity is not just a problem in the United States. It has become a global pandemic. According to the WHO, childhood obesity is prevalent around the world, particularly in urban areas in low- and middle-income countries. Worldwide, an estimated 22 million children age five or younger were overweight in 2007.

In order to combat childhood obesity, many health officials and policy makers

Michelle Obama on Obesity

Obesity is also one of the biggest threats to the American economy. If we continue on our current path, in ten years, nearly 50 percent of all Americans will be obese—not just overweight, but obese. So think about how much we'll be spending on health care to treat obesity-related conditions like heart disease, cancer, and diabetes. . . . And think about what this means for our quality of life—for how people feel when they wake up in the morning; whether they can make it through a day of work; whether they can do something as simple as walking to the store, or playing ball with their kids and grandkids. . . .

I know that achieving all this won't be easy—and it won't be quick. . . . But make no mistake about it, this problem can be solved.

We don't need to wait for some new invention or discovery to make this happen. This doesn't require fancy tools or technologies. We have everything we need right now—we have the information; we have the ideas; and we have the desire to start solving America's childhood obesity problem. The only question is whether we have the will.[5]

—Michelle Obama

An overweight teenage girl undergoes weekly tests to monitor her health.

are advocating for nutrition and physical education to better address obesity in schools. School lunch programs are of particular concern. Although many schools have banned soda in school cafeterias, other items sold in cafeterias remain high in fat and sugar. Chocolate milk, for example, contains as much sugar as the banned sodas. Federally subsidized school lunches are also typically made up of such items as chicken nuggets, french fries, and pizza, as opposed to healthier items such as grilled chicken, salad greens, and fresh fruits.

SOCIETY RESPONDS

Individuals and communities around the world rally against the growing obesity pandemic. Weight-loss aids and medical procedures have become a multibillion-dollar business as people seek ways to lose weight. Communities have started programs aimed at encouraging people to eat healthier and exercise more. Some governments have passed laws requiring restaurants to post nutritional information about their food.

Many people, however, continue to resist the public policies aimed at fighting the obesity pandemic. Some, particularly in the United States, consider the government's efforts in this area intrusive and an affront to personal freedoms. They do not feel the government should interfere in their personal decisions. Attempts by some local governments to add a sin tax to high-fat or sugary foods are often met with opposition. Proposed soda taxes, for example, would help generate income for state governments while also discouraging the consumption of sugary beverages that contribute to weight gain and obesity. However, many people resent the idea of the government attempting to influence their behavior in such a way.

Harvard economics professor N. Gregory Mankiw hypothesizes about such an approach:

> *Taxing soda may encourage better nutrition and benefit our future selves. But so could taxing candy, ice cream and fried foods. Subsidizing broccoli, gym memberships and dental floss comes next. Taxing mindless television shows and subsidizing serious literature cannot be far behind.* [6]

In addition, because of the new focus on the obesity pandemic, obese individuals sometimes find themselves targets of discrimination. Studies show that obese individuals make less money and have been promoted less often in the workplace than their slimmer counterparts. They may be ridiculed and ostracized. They are also sometimes financially penalized for their size, as in the case of airlines charging them for two seats.

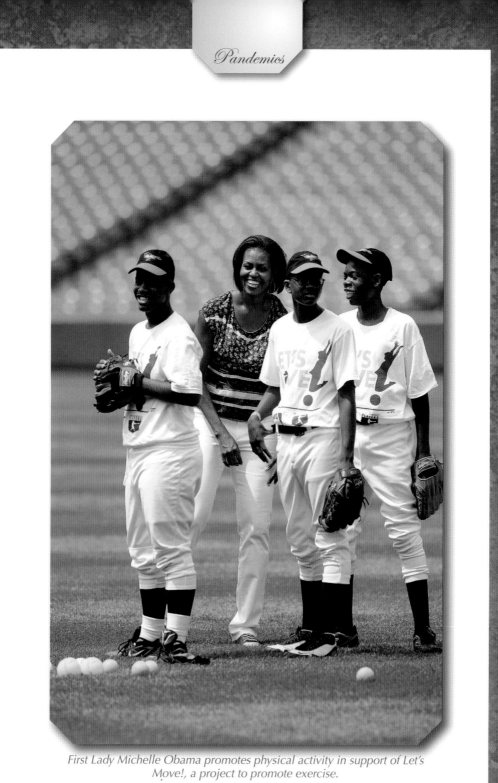

First Lady Michelle Obama promotes physical activity in support of Let's Move!, a project to promote exercise.

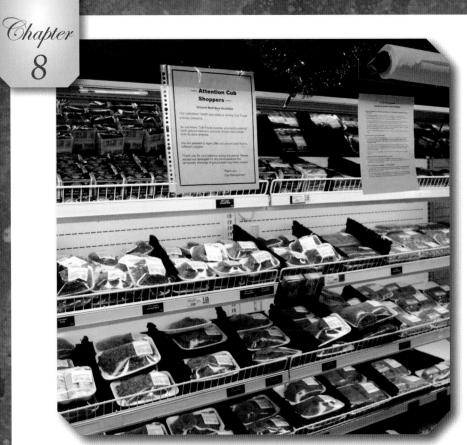

A notice informs customers of recalled ground beef products due to possible E. coli contamination.

Food–Borne Pandemics

n late 2009, most people's health concerns centered on the H1N1 influenza virus. But the US Department of Agriculture was worried about possible outbreaks from other pathogens. The federal agency issued recalls on several beef and ham products. They were concerned that these food items could be contaminated with Listeria, E. coli, or salmonella. Recalls are one of the most important tools that the government and public health officials have to fight off food-borne illnesses. It helps them get contaminated food out of the nation's supply before it has been consumed.

Government intervention is important because food-borne illnesses remain a serious threat even in the twenty-first century. Many of the pathogens that contaminate food, such as E. coli and salmonella, come from animals. Others, such as calicivirus, are passed from person to person when infected individuals handle food. According to the CDC, an estimated 76 million cases of food-borne disease occur annually in the United States. Although most cases are mild, 325,000 cases require hospitalization, and approximately

Typhoid Mary

Mary Mallon has the unfortunate fate to be known throughout history as "Typhoid Mary."

Mallon, who was born in Ireland in 1869, immigrated to the United States as a teenager. She worked as a cook for elite New York City families. She infected at least 47 people, three of whom died, with typhoid through handling food. Public health officials deemed her a threat to society and forcibly quarantined her for 26 years. However, Mary had no symptoms of the disease herself. She has since been identified as the first healthy carrier for typhoid. It is likely that she was born with the disease. Mallon's case shows the complexity of public health laws, science, and medicine along with the balance between individual rights and the government's right to protect its citizens.

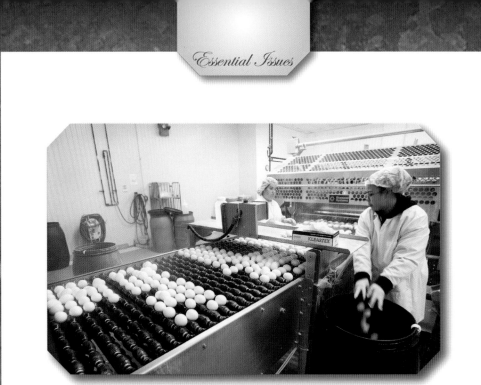

Pasteurizing eggs can help prevent the spread of food-borne illness.

5,000 of those cases are fatal. Food-borne illness is most serious among the very old, the very young, and people who are already sick. It can also be serious in healthy individuals who have consumed a large amount of the contaminate.

Food and Disease through History

Like other pandemic diseases, food-borne illnesses have been present throughout history. In the nineteenth century, typhoid fever was a serious threat. Typhoid fever is a bacterial infection that causes fever, headache, rash, and digestive problems. Patients with typhoid fever became weak and susceptible to other diseases. The fatality rate was approximately 10 percent. Cholera, which was once pandemic, could also be transmitted via contaminated food.

But much changed in the twentieth century. Advances in how food is produced and distributed, along with a better understanding of the microorganisms that cause disease, helped conquer some of history's worst food-borne illnesses. Technologies made food safer. For example, the process of pasteurizing, or heating, milk to kill disease-causing pathogens before it is sold to consumers became widespread in the twentieth century. And doctors and clinical laboratories are now required to report food-borne illnesses to government agencies. These reports have helped to contain diseases sooner than in the past.

Who Was Louis Pasteur?

Louis Pasteur was one of the founders of the field of microbiology. A French biologist, chemist, administrator, and educator, Pasteur made numerous contributions to the field of science during the mid- to late 1800s. After becoming a professor, he studied the process of fermentation. This work led to his theories about germs: specifically that food can contain microorganisms that can spoil food and sicken people. His experiments with fermentation also showed that heating liquids kills the microorganisms. This process could be applied to perishable fluids, such as milk, to keep them from spoiling and sickening people. This process is called pasteurization in his honor and is still used today for nearly all commercial milk products. He also developed vaccines for several deadly infections, including rabies, cholera, and anthrax.

However, some changes in the way food is produced and distributed created problems too. Refrigeration, which keeps foods from spoiling, also enables the growth of some microbes, such as Listeria. Mass production also means that when there is an outbreak, it can be widespread and affect many more people than it would have 100 years ago. In the past, many food-borne illnesses were locally contained. For example, if a family ate beets that were improperly canned at home, which was a common cause of botulism poisoning, they

Common Causes of Food-Borne Diseases

The CDC lists the following bacteria and viruses as the most common causes of food-borne diseases in the United States:

- Campylobacter: This bacterium is found on most raw poultry meat. People become sick when they eat undercooked chicken or food that has been contaminated with juices dripped from raw chicken. It causes fever, diarrhea, and abdominal cramps.
- Salmonella: This bacterium lives in the intestines of birds, reptiles, and mammals. People get it from eating undercooked meat that contains the bacteria. It can cause fever, diarrhea, and abdominal cramps. It can cause life-threatening infections if it invades the bloodstream.
- E. coli: This bacterium comes mostly from cattle. People become sick when they eat or drink the contaminated product and usually suffer severe, bloody diarrhea and painful abdominal cramps. E. coli can be fatal.
- Calicivirus or Norwalk-like virus: The virus is thought to spread from an infected person to another when the infected individual handles food. It can cause acute gastrointestinal illness; most people suffer vomiting.

would most likely be the only ones to become sick.

New food-borne diseases have also emerged. Concern about eating beef swept around the world in the late twentieth century after multiple cases of mad cow disease occurred in England. Mad cow disease causes the deterioration of the human brain. It is found in cattle; only in rare cases has it infected humans. The emergence of this disease set off economic and political reactions. Certain countries banned beef imports, and the value of cattle on the world economic markets tumbled.

The Cost of Being Sick

The US Department of Agriculture Economic Research Service calculated that each year food-borne diseases generate $6.9 billion in medical costs, lost productivity, and premature deaths. This figure does not account for additional costs, including the cost to travel to medical treatments, lost work time of those caring for the sick, or any emotional costs associated with the illness.

The Battle Continues

Victims of food-borne illnesses usually turn to their doctors or hospital emergency rooms for treatment. But the fight against these diseases does not end there. Public health departments monitor cases of food-borne illnesses. Local officials take the first reports, which are then submitted to state public health departments and passed on to the CDC.

Controversy over Irradiated Food

Technological advances have frequently been used to stop the spread of infectious diseases, but not all advances are welcome by everyone. Such is the case with irradiated food. Irradiation is a process by which food, including meat, is exposed to radiation to kill bacteria, parasites, mold, and fungi. Irradiated foods have been sold in the United States since 1992 but have not been widely available. Proponents say irradiation is an effective way to keep food safe, but others question its safety, saying that it has not been proven safe with long-term studies and that it could cause cancer.

Federal agencies also have the power to order food companies to recall products that are or could possibly be contaminated.

Although many countries have similar processes to monitor and report food-borne illnesses, global health officials also monitor for such things. At the beginning of 2010, the WHO promoted the idea of a "global strategy for the surveillance of food-borne diseases."[1] It wanted member states to set up laboratories to monitor both outbreaks and individual cases. The labs could also check food for chemicals and microorganisms.

The WHO advocates for improved research into the causes and spread of food-borne disease. With more research and a better understanding of food-borne illness, doctors and governments will be better prepared to respond to problems regarding food-borne disease and food contamination.

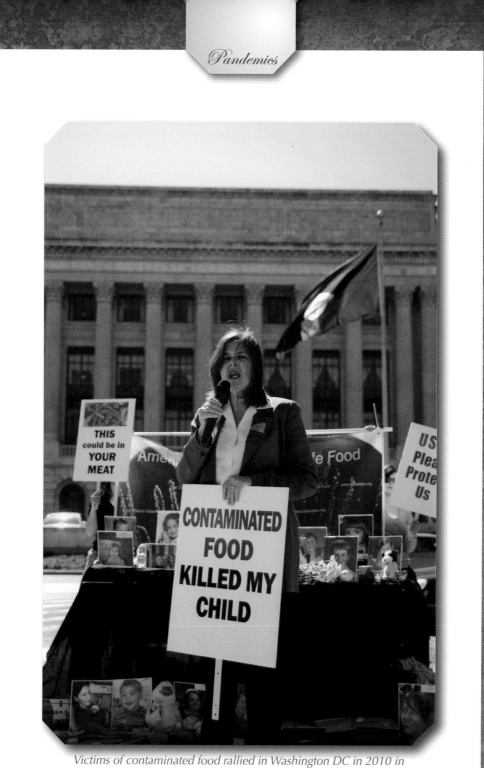

Victims of contaminated food rallied in Washington DC in 2010 in support of stricter measures in food production.

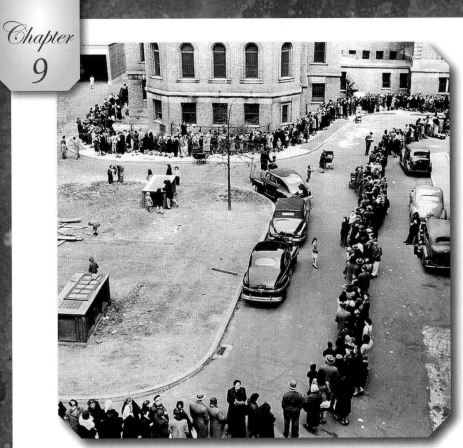

People lined up outside Morrisania Hospital in New York in 1947 to receive smallpox vaccinations.

THE FIGHT CONTINUES

eginning in the 1950s, WHO officials began to battle the kinds of diseases that caused pandemics. They established vaccination programs and carried out pest elimination projects to cut down on the diseases rodents carried. They implemented reporting programs to track and investigate outbreaks. And they teamed up with government and nongovernmental organizations and private foundations in their fight against a number of diseases, such as polio and HIV/AIDS.

As part of the efforts to control and prevent pandemics, WHO officials want to know about outbreaks before they spread. To that end, it has established a Global Outbreak Alert and Response Network (GOARN). WHO member nations, which have agreed to work toward public health under the WHO, report when cases of the diseases covered by the network are discovered. The diseases covered include avian influenza, bubonic plague, and smallpox.

New Diseases Emerge

Despite efforts from the WHO and others on the front lines of public health, the world is not safe from diseases capable of becoming pandemics. As the 2009 H1N1 pandemic proved, the influenza virus

Destroying the Last Smallpox Virus

The United States and Russia hold the last two remaining samples of the smallpox virus. Officials have not destroyed them because these samples could be needed for scientific research. But others fear the samples could lead to the creation of a bioterrorist weapon or accidental exposure to the disease—both of which could lead to a pandemic among the world's population that is now largely unvaccinated against smallpox. As of 2010, both samples still existed.

remains capable of becoming a pandemic without much warning.

Other human diseases continue to appear, though many of the most devastating diseases that once plagued human civilization are better controlled and more effectively treated today. Cholera has never gone away. And as of 2010, polio, a serious viral infection that attacks the brain and spinal cord, still occurs. In fact, the only disease to ever have been eradicated is smallpox, with the last known case occurring in 1977.

Rotary International Takes Up the Fight

Rotary International, a worldwide organization that provides humanitarian services and promotes peace, took up a global fight against polio in 1985. Its efforts, in part, led to the 1988 launch of the Global Polio Eradication Initiative. This initiative brings together the WHO, the United Nations Children's Fund (UNICEF), and the United States, along with Rotary International, in a massive effort to immunize children against polio and eradicate the disease.

Polio is a serious viral infection. It most often affects children under the age of five. The poliovirus attacks the brain and spinal cord. One of every 200 infected children becomes paralyzed. Of those cases, 5 to 10 percent die because their breathing muscles become paralyzed. A vaccine for polio was developed in the 1950s. Since then, polio has been eradicated in most developed nations. Many developing nations still experience polio outbreaks.

When the initiative started, polio was active in 125 countries and infected approximately 1,000 children every day. But according to the WHO, polio cases decreased by more than 99 percent between 1988 and 2006. By 2008, only four countries had polio cases. Those countries were Afghanistan, India, Nigeria, and Pakistan.

Still, new diseases are emerging. Some, such as HIV/AIDS, have already become pandemic. International organizations including the WHO, the International AIDS Society, AVERT, and UNAIDS are working to control the AIDS pandemic. They educate people about preventing HIV infection. They work to get treatment to people who need it. They promote research into finding new treatments for HIV/AIDS, and they hope to one day find a vaccine or cure for the disease.

In addition to fighting diseases that are already at pandemic levels, health organizations are watchful for disease that have the potential to become pandemics. One such example is the Ebola virus. The WHO called it "one of the most virulent viral diseases known to humankind."[1] It was first identified in 1976 in Sudan and Zaire (which was renamed the Democratic Republic of the Congo in 1997). Ebola causes death in 80 to 90 percent of those infected. The virus is spread when someone has direct contact with the blood, body fluids, or tissues of an infected person. It can also be spread by handling animals, including chimpanzees, gorillas, and monkeys that have the disease.

Occasional deadly outbreaks of Ebola have been occurring in Africa since the 1970s. Prevention efforts include educating the public about transmission and quarantining infected individuals. There is no cure or vaccine. However, researchers are working on the problem of treating Ebola. In 2010, a Boston University research team announced that it had successful trials in preventing the virus in monkeys. A drug for humans might one day help contain outbreaks in Africa.

SARS is another example of an emerging disease with pandemic potential. SARS, or Severe Acute Respiratory Syndrome, emerged in China in late 2002. By early 2003, it had spread to 25 other countries in Asia, the Americas, and Europe. SARS is characterized by high fever, coughing, and difficulty breathing. In severe cases, this is followed by pneumonia and respiratory failure. Approximately 6 percent of those infected die.

Alarmed by the outbreak of this new disease, the WHO and the CDC began research into its cause and established measures to contain it. They issued reports and updates for doctors and public health officials around the world and urged that airline passengers be screened for symptoms.

Most treatments, including antibiotics, steroids, and antiviral drugs, are ineffective against SARS. Scientists soon discovered that SARS was a form of coronavirus. These viruses typically cause common colds in humans. The SARS coronavirus, however, is unrelated to those that cause colds in humans. Scientists believe the SARS virus came from bats. Because coronaviruses had not been threatening to humans, little research had been done to discover antiviral drugs that would treat infections. In 2004, Chinese scientists reported the development of an effective vaccine against SARS. However, by the time the vaccine was ready for distribution, the outbreak had subsided and the vaccine was never used. Approximately 350 people in China had already died from SARS. The emergence of a new disease requires scientists to act quickly to discover effective treatments and vaccines. However, in the case of a rapidly spreading disease, science may be too slow to reach those who need help before an outbreak subsides.

"Safe drinking water and basic sanitation are intrinsic to human survival, well-being and dignity. . . . Each day, thousands of parents in the developing world are left to watch their children die from these wholly preventable causes. Their plight, their daily suffering, diminishes all of us and compels us to act."[2]
—Ban-Ki Moon,
United Nations
Secretary-General

LACK OF SANITATION

The lack of adequate water and sanitation facilities remained a problem at the beginning of the twenty-first century. The WHO estimates that approximately 1.1 billion people in the world do not have access to clean water. An additional 2.4 billion people do not have access to adequate sanitation facilities. Approximately 2 million people, mostly children younger than five years of age, die every year due to diarrhea-related diseases.

The United Nations prioritized clean drinking water as one of its Millennium Development Goals in 2001. Its goal is to halve the number of people without access to safe drinking water and sanitation by 2015. Other organizations, such as England's Water Aid, work with communities in Africa and Asia to establish clean sources of drinking water and sanitation close to home. They also work with government leaders and policy makers to ensure that the government makes clean drinking water and sanitation a priority.

THE HUMAN THREAT

At the start of the twenty-first century, government and public health officials feared that one of the biggest threats of another pandemic came from humans in the form of bioterrorism. The CDC defined bioterrorism as "the deliberate release of viruses, bacteria, or other germs (agents) used to cause illness or death in people, animals, or plants."[3]

In the early twenty-first century, with the United States engaged in wars in the Middle East, government leaders and policy makers believed that the United States was vulnerable to bioterrorism. In 2001, letters containing anthrax, a powerful bacterial disease, were sent anonymously through the US mail to various businesses and government offices. The attacks killed five people.

The potential for other bioterrorist attacks caused public concern. Contamination of the food or water supply could cause many US citizens to become ill. Airborne toxins could also be devastating. Diseases that could be used by terrorists include cholera, bubonic plague, and smallpox, among others. These diseases could spread quickly. And because they rarely occur naturally in the United States, hospitals and medical centers would be unable to treat a large number of infected individuals.

Government and world leaders prepare to protect the world against these possible pandemics just as officials around the world prepare to fight naturally occurring pandemic diseases.

PANDEMICS CONTINUE

The human population remains vulnerable to disease. Despite many advances in medical technology, including treatments and vaccines against many deadly diseases, illness and disease continue to spread. Viruses and bacteria that cause disease mutate, making some drugs ineffective at treating infection. And with global travel, disease is more easily spread across the world.

In many developing nations, people lack clean living conditions and access to medical care. People there are especially vulnerable to illness and outbreaks of deadly diseases.

When an outbreak begins, it is difficult to predict just how easily the disease will spread or how deadly it will be. But scientists and government officials must prepare for the worst. They must respond quickly to outbreaks if they are to prevent the spread of dangerous communicable disease and protect public health.

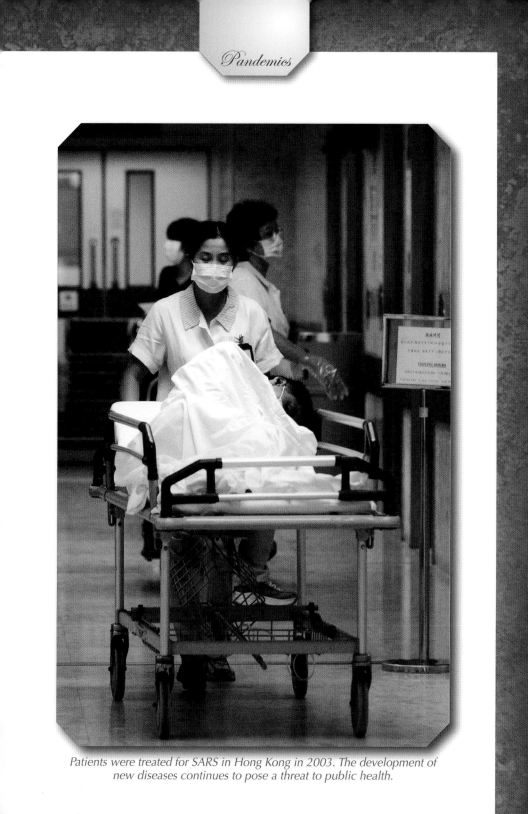

Patients were treated for SARS in Hong Kong in 2003. The development of new diseases continues to pose a threat to public health.

TIMELINE

1338	1495	1798
The bubonic plague pandemic begins.	Syphilis sweeps through Europe, starting a pandemic of the disease.	British physician Edward Jenner successfully vaccinates people against smallpox.

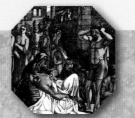

1918	1945	1947
The 1918 influenza pandemic occurs.	The United Nations is founded.	The World Health Organization (WHO) is formed.

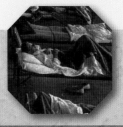

1826

A major cholera pandemic begins in India.

1832

European immigrants bring cholera to Canada.

1849

Dr. John Snow publishes a paper suggesting that cholera is spread by contaminated water.

1952

The WHO organizes the Global Influenza Surveillance Network.

1957

Asian influenza spreads from China, causing a pandemic.

1968

Hong Kong influenza emerges out of China and spreads around the world.

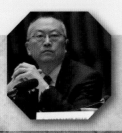

TIMELINE

1976	1977	1981
Researchers identify the Ebola virus, a deadly emerging disease, in Africa.	The last known case of naturally occurring smallpox occurs in Somalia.	The CDC publishes a brief clinical report on a rare pneumonia. It is the first sign of the emerging AIDS pandemic.

1997	2002	2004
The deadly avian influenza emerges in Asia.	SARS, or Severe Acute Respiratory Syndrome, emerges in China.	In May, the WHO issues its Global Strategy on Diet, Physical Activity, and Health.

1983

American and
French researchers
identify the virus
that causes AIDS.

1985

Rotary International,
a civic group, takes
up a global fight
against polio.

1988

The WHO spearheads
the launch of
the Global Polio
Eradication Initiative.

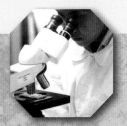

2007

On February 1, the
US Department of
Health and Human
Services unveils new
efforts to advance
pandemic influenza
preparedness.

2009

Dr. Margaret Chan,
the director-general
of the WHO, declares
an H1N1 influenza
pandemic on June 11.

2010

One billion adults
are overweight.

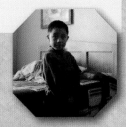

ESSENTIAL FACTS

AT ISSUE

❖ Some of the germs that cause diseases can change over time. This means humans are constantly vulnerable to disease. These mutations also make predicting the potential for a pandemic more difficult.

❖ AIDS first emerged in the United States in 1981, but cases in other countries quickly followed. Scientists raced to develop effective treatments, but still did not have a vaccine or a cure as of 2010.

❖ Obesity has become a pandemic in the late twentieth century. Although genetic and biological factors play a part in obesity, high-fat foods, too much food, and little exercise contribute significantly.

❖ Modern food production and distribution have played a part in food-borne illnesses, as mass-produced food could be capable of sickening many people in large geographical areas.

CRITICAL DATES

1300s
The bubonic plague pandemic, or the Black Death, wiped out major portions of the population in Europe.

1798
British physician Edward Jenner successfully vaccinated people against smallpox.

1918
Spanish influenza spreads across the globe.

1947
The World Health Organization (WHO) was formed, and five years later it organized the Global Influenza Surveillance Network.

June 5, 1981
The US Centers for Disease Control and Prevention published a brief clinical report on a rare pneumonia. It was the first sign of the emerging AIDS pandemic.

June 11, 2009
Dr. Margaret Chan, the director-general of WHO, declared an H1N1 influenza pandemic.

QUOTES

"No previous pandemic has been detected so early or watched so closely, in real-time, right at the very beginning. The world can now reap the benefits of investments, over the last five years, in pandemic preparedness. We have a head start. This places us in a strong position. But it also creates a demand for advice and reassurance in the midst of limited data and considerable scientific uncertainty."—*WHO announcement from Dr. Margaret Chan, June 11, 2009*

"Safe drinking water and basic sanitation are intrinsic to human survival, well-being and dignity. . . . Each day, thousands of parents in the developing world are left to watch their children die from these wholly preventable causes. Their plight, their daily suffering, diminishes all of us and compels us to act."—*Ban-Ki Moon, United Nations Secretary-General*

GLOSSARY

anesthesiologist
A doctor who specializes in administering anesthetics.

communicable
Capable of being transmitted.

epidemic
Widespread occurrence of a disease.

epidemiologist
A scientist who tracks diseases and studies epidemics.

exponentially
Having an exponential, or very high, growth rate.

genetic
Pertaining to or produced by genes.

hemophilia
A hereditary, potentially fatal disorder in which blood fails to clot.

intravenous
Administered or injected into a vein by a needle.

median
The middle value in a list of numerically arranged values. In the set 3, 7, 14, 36, 48, the median is 14.

microbe
A microscopic organism, such as a bacterium, often responsible for disease.

mortality rate
The percentage of victims who die from a particular disease.

mutate
To change or alter.

obstetrician
A doctor who specializes in obstetrics, or the care of women during pregnancy and childbirth.

organism
> A life form.

outbreak
> Sudden occurrence of disease in an area.

pathogen
> A disease-producing agent.

reproduce
> To produce again; to replicate or copy.

strain
> A microorganism with a distinct form.

toxin
> A chemical or substance that is harmful to the body and can cause illness.

venereal disease
> A disease that is spread through sexual contact.

virulent
> Intensively noxious or poisonous.

ADDITIONAL RESOURCES

SELECTED BIBLIOGRAPHY

Dudley, William. (Editor). *Epidemics: Opposing Viewpoints*. San Diego: Greenhaven Press. 1999.

Marks, Geoffrey and William K Beatty. *Epidemics*. New York: Charles Scribner's Sons. 1976.

Oldstone, Michael B.A. *Viruses, Plagues, & History*. New York: Oxford University Press, 1988.

Snodgrass, Mary Ellen. *World Epidemics: A Cultural Chronology of Disease from Prehistory to the Era of SARS*. Jefferson, NC: McFarland & Company. 2003.

Youngman, Barry. *Pandemics and Global Health*. New York: Infobase. 2008.

FURTHER READINGS

Barnard, Bryn. *Outbreak! Plagues That Changed History*. New York: Crown Books for Young Readers. 2005.

Bollet, Alfred Jay. *Plagues & Poxes*. New York: Demos Medical Publishing, 2004.

Goldsmith, Connie. *Influenza: The Next Pandemic?* New York: Twenty-First Century Books. 2006.

Grady, Denise. *New York Times Deadly Invaders: Virus Outbreaks Around The World, from Marburn Fever to Avian Flu*. Boston: Kingfisher Publications. 2006.

Web Links

To learn more about pandemics, visit ABDO Publishing Company on the World Wide Web at **www.abdopublishing.com**. Web sites about pandemics are featured on our Book Links page. These links are routinely monitored and updated to provide the most current information available.

For More Information

For more information on this subject, contact or visit the following organizations.

US Centers for Disease Control and Prevention
1600 Clifton Road, Atlanta, GA 30333
800-232-4636
www.cdc.gov
The CDC works to protect public health in the United States.

US National Institutes of Health
9000 Rockville Pike, Bethesda, MD 20892
301-496-4000
www.nih.gov
The NIH is a US government agency responsible for researching diseases and other health issues.

World Health Organization
Avenue Appia 20, 1211 Geneva 27, Switzerland
41-22-791-21-11
www.who.int
The WHO coordinates international responses to public health crises.

SOURCE NOTES

Chapter 1. A New Threat

1. "World Now at the Start of 2009 Influenza Pandemic." *who. int*. World Health Organization, 11 Jun. 2009. Web. 4 Jan. 2010.

2. Charles Holmes. "Swine Flu Prompts a World of Different Reactions." *npr.org*. National Public Radio. 29 Apr. 2009. Web. 4 Jan. 2010.

3. "World Now at the Start of 2009 Influenza Pandemic." *who. int*. World Health Organization, 11 Jun. 2009. Web. 4 Jan. 2010.

4. Charles Holmes. "Swine Flu Prompts a World of Different Reactions." *npr.org*. National Public Radio. 29 Apr. 2009. Web. 4 Jan. 2010.

5. Ibid.

6. "Paranoia Pandemic: Conservative Media Baselessly Blame Swine Flu Outbreak on Immigrants." *mediamatters.org*. Media Matters for America, 27 Apr. 2009. Web. 4 Jan. 2010.

Chapter 2. What Is a Pandemic?

1. Lawrence K. Altman. "The Doctor's World: Is This a Pandemic? Define 'Pandemic.'" *New York Times Online*. 9 Jun. 2009. Web. 4 Jan. 2010.

2. "Global Alert and Response." *who.int*. World Health Organization, 11 Jun. 2009. Web. 4 Jan. 2010.

3. Ibid.

4. "Health Experts: Obesity Pandemic Looms." *msnbc.com*. MSNBC, 3 Sept. 2006. Web. 4 Jan. 2010.

Chapter 3. What Causes a Pandemic?

1. "Global Alert and Response/Pandemic Preparedness." *who. int*. World Health Organization, 11 Jun. 2009. Web. 4 Jan. 2010

Chapter 4. A History of Pandemics
None.

Chapter 5. Influenza Today
None.

Chapter 6. HIV/AIDS
1. "WHO and HIV/AIDS." *who.int*. World Health Organization, 11 Jun. 2009. Web. 4 Jan. 2009.

Chapter 7. The Rise of the Obesity Pandemic
1. "Obesity and Overweight." *who.int*. World Health Organization, 11 Jun. 2009. Web. 4 Jan. 2009.

2. "Overweight and Obesity." *cdc.gov*. Centers for Disease Control and Prevention, 11 Jun. 2009. Web. 4 Jan. 2009.

3. Josie Raymond. "Surgeon General Says Obesity a Result of Poor Choices." healthcare.change.org. *Change.org*, 3 Feb. 2010. Web. 28 Jul. 2010.

4. "The Surgeon General's Call to Action to Prevent and Decrease Overweight and Obesity." *surgeongeneral.gov*. Department of Health and Human Services, 13 Dec. 2001. Web. 4 Jan. 2010.

5. Michelle Obama. "Obesity Is Also One of the Biggest Threats to the American Economy." *Chicago Sun Times Online*, 20 Jan. 2010. Web. 29 Jul. 2010

6. N. Gregory Mankiw. "Can a Soda Tax Save Us From Ourselves?" *New York Times Online*, 6 Jun. 2010. Web. 27 Aug 2010.

SOURCE NOTES CONTINUED

Chapter 8. Food-Borne Pandemics

1. "General Information Related to Foodborne Disease." *who. int*. World Health Organization, 11 Jun. 2009. Web. 4 Jan. 2010.

Chapter 9. The Fight Continues

1. "Global Alert and Response/Ebola Haemorrhagic Fever." *who.int*. World Health Organization, 11 Jun. 2009. Web. 4 Jan. 2010.

2. Alina Haddad. "Ban Ki-moon Addresses Water Scarcity and Sanitation." *mediaglobal.org*. Media Global: Voices of the Global South, 28 Sept. 2008. Web. 28 Jul. 2010.

3. "Emergency Preparedness and Response." *bt.cdc.gov*. Centers for Disease Control and Prevention, 11 Jun. 2009. Web. 4 Jan. 2010.

INDEX

INDEX

ABOUT THE AUTHOR

Mary K. Pratt is a freelance journalist based in Massachusetts. She writes for a variety of publications, including newspapers, magazines, and trade journals. She has covered topics ranging from business to technology. She has won several awards, including a 1998 Primary Care Journalism Award and a 1998 first-place features award from the New England Press Association News Executives Association.

PHOTO CREDITS